Antonio Solini

Atlas of Automated Percutaneous Lumbar Discectomy (A.P.L.D.)
According to the Onik Method

Consulting Editor: Gary Onik
Translator: Sylvia Notini

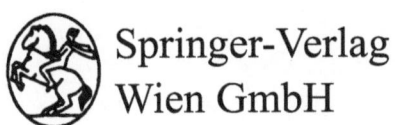 Springer-Verlag
Wien GmbH

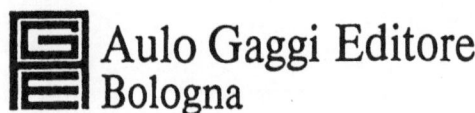 Aulo Gaggi Editore
Bologna

Antonio Solini, M.D.

Head, Department of Orthopaedics and Traumatology,
Hospital Molinette, Turin, Italy

Gary Onik, M.D.

Interventional Radiologist,
Allegheny-Singer Research Institute, Pittsburgh, Pa., U.S.A.

Sylvia Notini, Ph. D.

Professor at the University, Bologna, Italy

Translation from the Italian edition
Atlante della Nuclectomia Percutanea (secondo Onik)
© 1989 by Aulo Gaggi Editore, Bologna

ISBN 978-3-7091-3334-7   ISBN 978-3-7091-3332-3 (eBook)
DOI 10.1007/978-3-7091-3332-3

With 59 mostly coloured Figures (199 single illustrations)

Index

Preface

This text is an atlas: it is not a complete treatise on the development and maturation of this method, which the author has already seen to (G. Onik and Clyde A. Helms: Automated percutaneous lumbar discectomy. Radiology Research and Education Foundation. S. Francisco CA., 1988).

Nor is it meant to report our personal series of cases, however numerous they may be, a study which was begun in June 1987, and which was dealt with in many journals and publications on orthopaedics.

An atlas must essentially be descriptive and practical: we set this goal for ourselves, and hope to have achieved it.

I have tried to provide the reader who wishes to begin using this method with a succession of its various stages. I have extensively dealt with all indications for use.

It was not difficult for me to put this text-atlas together; I enjoyed the work, enthusiastically supported by my great love for orthopaedics and for anything that may bring improvement to the field. I am not a staunch upholder of new methods, rather I am a critical observer and an accurate evaluater of any innovation; what is «new» is not in itself either good or bad. An honest and thoughtful surgeon must evaluate the results, as they are the only witness of the reliability of a method.

Percutaneous discectomy according to the Onik method has all of the requirements: however, it cannot as yet be evaluated in time.

It has been said of the Codivilla operation for congenital talipes equinovarus that it was perfect from the very start and as such cannot be improved. This is not so for the Onik method.

Time will certainly be a good judge.

Controversy arose as I began to use the method: the fact that I personally discussed the method with Gary Onik, that we extensively discussed the advantages and the disadvantages of the method, the fact that I personally absorbed the method and its aims, place me way above any diatribe.

I do not love the Onik method; I use it in a select number of cases. I will judge it in the future.

I wish to thank my collaborators: Dr. Gabriele Orsini and Dr. Bruno Paschero who truly contributed to the writing of the text: these are faithful and mature men, as well as competent and prepared technicians.

I would also like to thank Mr. Maurizio Tresoldi, a life-long friend and an expert photographer who greatly contributed to the illustrations in the atlas.

Finally, I wish to thank Prof. Gianfranco Fineschi who benevolently wished to present our work; no one better than he, the father of disc herniation surgery in Italy, could have done it. His esteem honors us, and encourages us to proceed in our study of the pathology of the vertebral column.
Turin, October 1988

PROF. ANTONIO SOLINI

Preface to the English edition

Percutaneous discectomy originated with the work of Dr. Hijikata in Tokyo who showed that percutaneous disc removal through a cannula with a pituitary Rondeur could affect long-term relief of sciatic pain. Since his original work, a number of other investigators using basically the same approach have confirmed the results. Percutaneous discectomy, however, has limited theoretical value if the morbidity associated with the procedure is not low. Recent literature, however, has shown that this hand method of percutaneous discectomy can be associated with significant morbidity including major vessel damage, nerve damage, and a high rate of discitis.

The concept of automated percutaneous discectomy was to decrease the size of the instrumentation markedly, while still allowing rapid disc removal, therefore decreasing tissue trauma and decreasing the chances of complications. Equally important as the small instrumentation was the development of a procedure with a strong emphasis on radiographic landmarks and visualization, which this book faithfully describes in an excellent manner.

The incorporation of a new procedure into general medical practice has a number of steps beyond the initial idea, the making of the equipment, and the first series of patients. Critical to the success of any new procedure is its application and validation by other surgeons outside the original group of investigators. Dr. Solini was one of the first Europeans to recognize the possible importance of this procedure and the first Italian physician to come to Pittsburgh to learn the procedure.

The subsequent study that he and the other Italian investigators published, reproduced the results of our original study and has helped establish the procedure.

The next critical step beyond this is the confirmation that the procedure is safe and effective in the hands of practicing physicians in the community who are not investigators. The procedure has now been performed over 35,000 times, and there is still no documented instance of great vessel damage, permanent nerve injury, or intraoperative death, showing that it may be safely practiced in the community.

Like all procedures, we are sure automated percutaneous discectomy will evolve over time as more is learned through experience. Despite this fact, the basic fundamentals of the procedure will remain the basis for the safe application of the procedure and therefore ensure this book's continued value in the future.

GARY ONIK, M.D.
University of Pittsburgh
1988

Foreword

This atlas is the product of a praiseworthy and original initiative.

Prof. Solini's personality characterizes the conceptual and organizational aspect of the text, and inspires the informative sequences that his collaborators were able to add to the study.

The authors, all of them, have shown their ability to exhibit proof of true competence (which only a few others, in Italy, are capable of possessing in equal measure) in an avant-garde subject such as this one.

This is a subject which still requires data and verification, which has many aspects that need defining, but which has already shown its positive results, results which, it may be stated, are destined to increase in the near future.

As may be said of every avant-garde subject, this material requires serious and well-organized study, clear diagnostic competence, an exact use of methodology. And the authors possess all of these elements.

By consulting their atlas, all of us, even those of us who are already familiar with the method, may learn. All of us may make use of the atlas, because every detail of the method is presented and illustrated.

Previous publications by Prof. Solini and his research group at the Division of Orthopaedics at the Molinette Hospital in Turin have provided data and testimony on their excellent work on this subject, and have convinced us of its efficacy.

For this reason I had no difficulty writing the introduction to the atlas.

PROF. GIANFRANCO FINESCHI

Introduction

N. Ruggieri

Methods for the percutaneous treatment of disc pathology were first applied after the introduction of techniques used for chemical herniectomy.

In 1961 Lymon Smith proposed treatment of intervertebral disc herniation by using a needle to intradiscally inject a chymopapain solution (proteolotic enzyme extracted from Carica Papaja) capable of chemically digesting the vertebral pulpy nucleus, the cause of neurological compression.

The initial enthusiastic diffusion of the method, which continued to be used extensively, was considerably mitigated when complications related to allergy (anaphylaxis) or neuroradicular deficit occured.

It is for this reason that there has been considerable support of methods of percutaneous herniectomy allowing for the removal of the disc nucleus without using chemical products, at the same time avoiding the drawbacks of a traditional open surgical or microsurgical approach.

In 1975 Hijikata devised a method of percutaneous approach to the disc which through a 5 mm cannula inserted as far as the posterior part of the anulus, allowed for its incision and the removal of the pulpy nucleus; this was done using special instruments devised for surgery of the hypophysary gland. The author reported having obtained good results in 80% of the patients thus treated.

Subsequently, other methods of this type were devised by Kambin (1983), and Suezava and Schreiber (1983, 1986).

In 85% of his cases, Kambin obtained good results by using Craig biopsy instrumentation under radioscopic monitoring to grasp and remove the herniated disc material with a large trocar type needle pointed at the anulus fibrosus.

Suezava and Schreiber, instead, used the instrumentation proposed by Hijikata, with some technical (a shaver was used to obtain more accurate toilet of the disc) and visual (the use of an optic fiber discoscope inserted contralaterally in the disc to monitor the progress of disc removal) modifications.

This method obtained good results even in cases of disc protrusion associated with lumbar stenotic compression.

Intraoperative staining of the disc with methylene blue was also proposed, to allow for better intraoperative visualization under the discoscope.

Furthermore, Jacobson proposed a method of lateral access to the disc; the author used a 10-11 mm diameter cannula under general anesthesia. Nonetheless, because of a high percentage of internal organ and peripheral nerve complications, Friedman used the method to conduct a study on cadavers, concluding that it appeared to be particularly dangerous.

In 1984 Gary Onik perfected a method of percutaneous discectomy, using an instrument which, in addition to being simple to use, was small in size, with a probe which was only 2 mm in diameter.

This recently applied method of discectomy makes use of an external vacuum suction mechanism to remove the disc chips, which are cut by a blade placed on the tip of the probe, in the manner of a guillotine, until the disc nucleus is completely empty.

The method is carried out under local anesthesia, with radioscopic and intraoperative discographic monitoring.

The method has obtained excellent results, with no complications, as long as the preliminary criteria established by the author are respected.

Clinical indications
N. Guercio

— **Protocol according to Maroon and Onik**
— **Clinical examination**
— **Psychoalgesimetric examination**

Protocol according to Maroon and Onik

The clinical evaluation is an essential phase in determining those patients who, after instrumental proof has been obtained, may be treated by percutaneous discectomy for disc pathology.

In order to avoid using procedures which are still at an experimental stage, it may be useful to emphasize just how important it is to respect all of the features expressed in the Maroon and Onik protocol, which essentially identify the case of contained disc protrusion characterized by lumbar pain and, in particular, sciatic pain symptoms, and precise nerve root involvement.

The first basic stage in a clinical evaluation of the case involves the gathering of a history of the patient, allowing for an identification of the existence of «risk» pathology (such as diabetes, lead poisoning, neoplasia, alcoholism, psychoneurosis, etc.) and for an exact definition of the typology, chronology, and of the entity of the symptoms, and of how they began, as well as of the topographical distribution of pain and sensory disorders.

A complete objective examination is then carried out, with particular regard for evidence of signs of disc pathology (antalgic scoliosis) and nerve root pathology (neurological deficit), so that clinical assessment may as accurately as possible diagnose the site of the disc pathology.

It is our belief that a psychoalgesimetric evaluation of the patients is also necessary, according to a protocol devised and currently in use at our Division for different types of pathology, in order to identify and, if necessary, exclude from treatment, those patients affected with psychological disorders involving important non-organic components, and which could influence the results of surgery, despite good anatomic and functional results.

PROTOCOL ACCORDING TO MAROON AND ONIK (1987)

1) Monolateral sciatic pain prevailing over lumbar pain.

2) Paresthesiae distributed over a precise dermatomeric area.

3) Positive Lasègue or Wasserman-Boschi sign.

4) Positive radiological signs specific for nerve root deficit.

5) Symptoms which for at least 6 weeks are unresponsive to conservative treatment.

6) Computerized tomographic confirmation of disc protrusion in the site of peripheral symptoms.

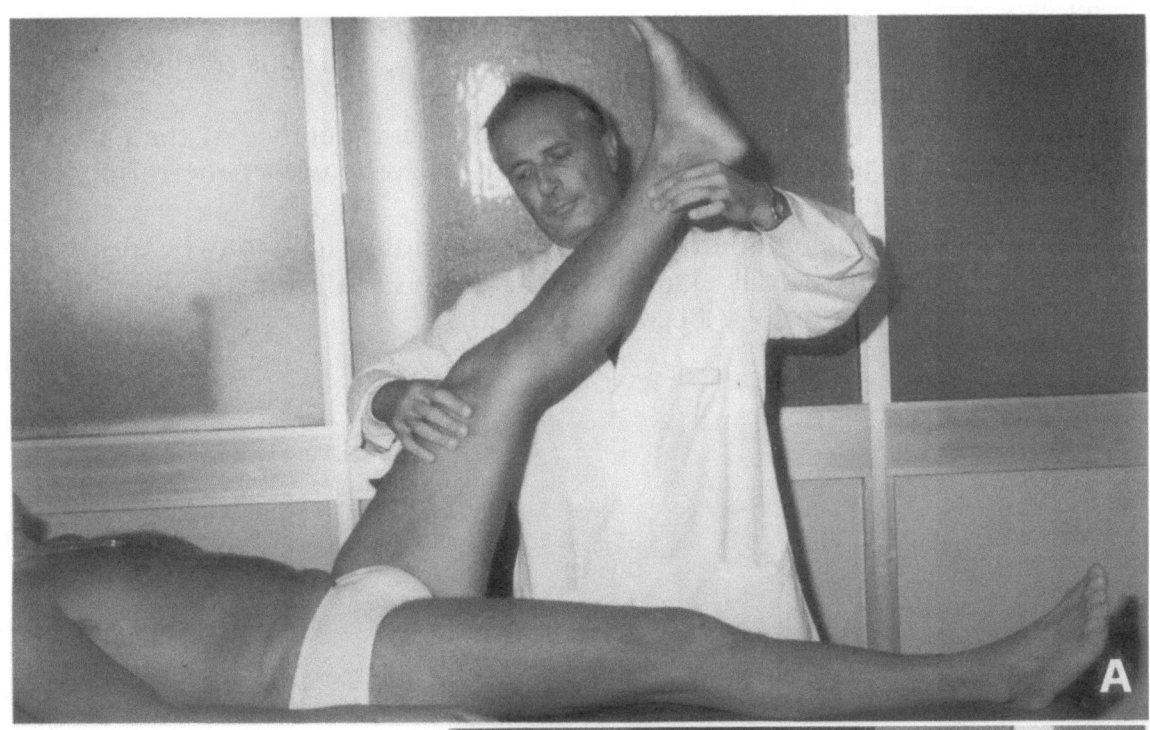

Clinical examination

The Lasègue sign (A), when there is sciatic pain, or the Wasserman-Boschi sign, when there is crural pain, must be positive on the side involved.

The presence of antalgic scoliosis (B) is always the expression of acute disc pathology.

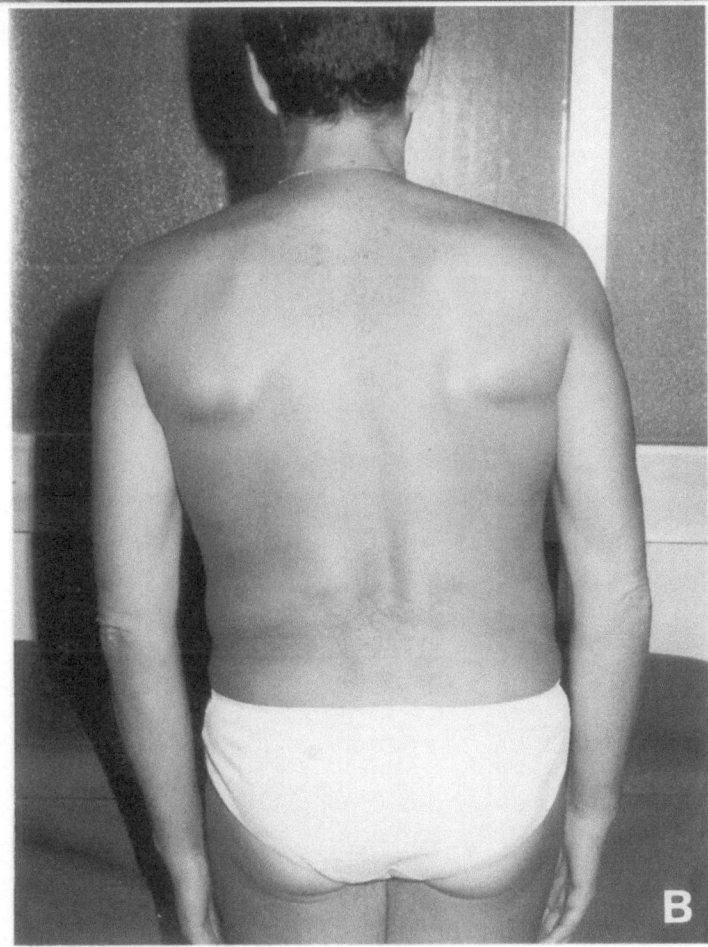

The weaking or absence of the patellar reflex (A) is to a greater or lesser extent an expression of pathology in the root of L_3, and thus of disc pathology between L_2 and L_3.

It must be kept in mind that the neurological competence of the patellar reflex is extended to the roots of L_2 and L_4, as well, with penetration depending on the individual case.

Hyposthenia of the tendon of the tibialis anterior, which may be observed at the ankle when the foot is extended (B) signifies pathology at the root of L_4 and, thus, disc pathology between L_3 and L_4.

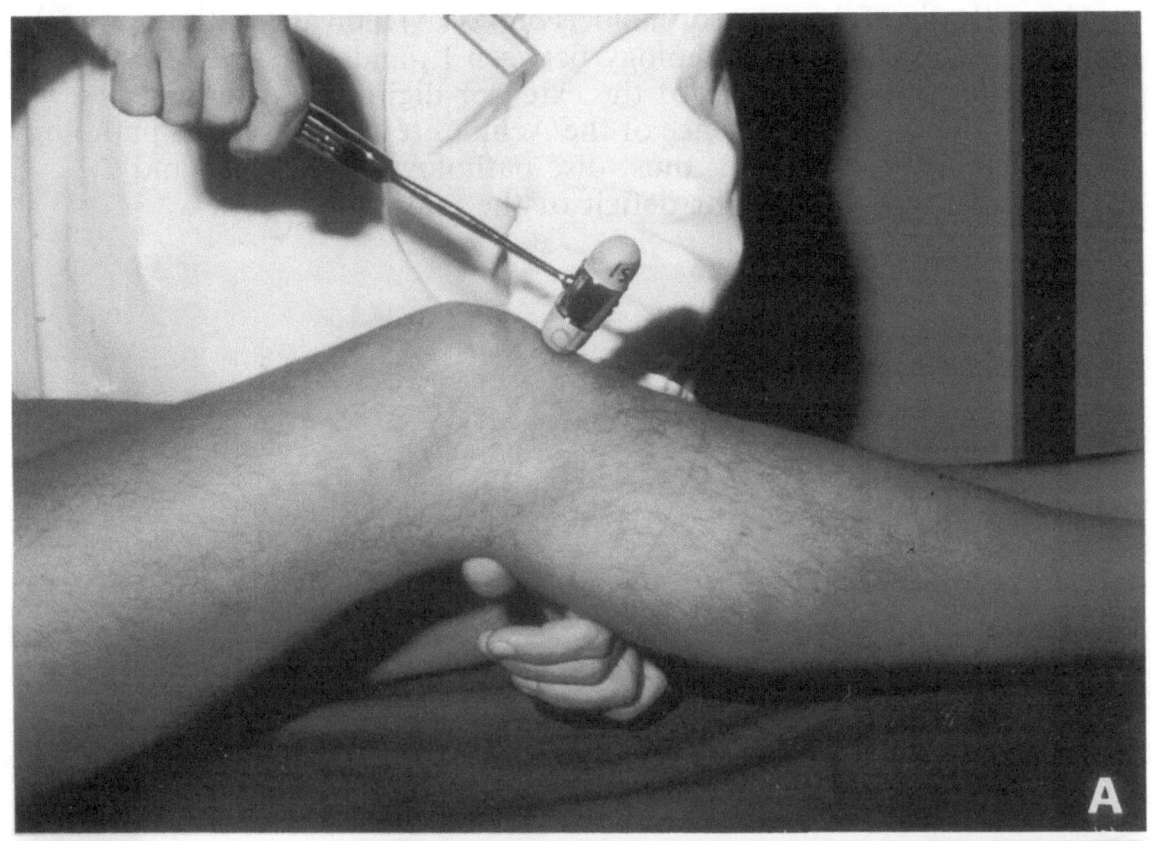

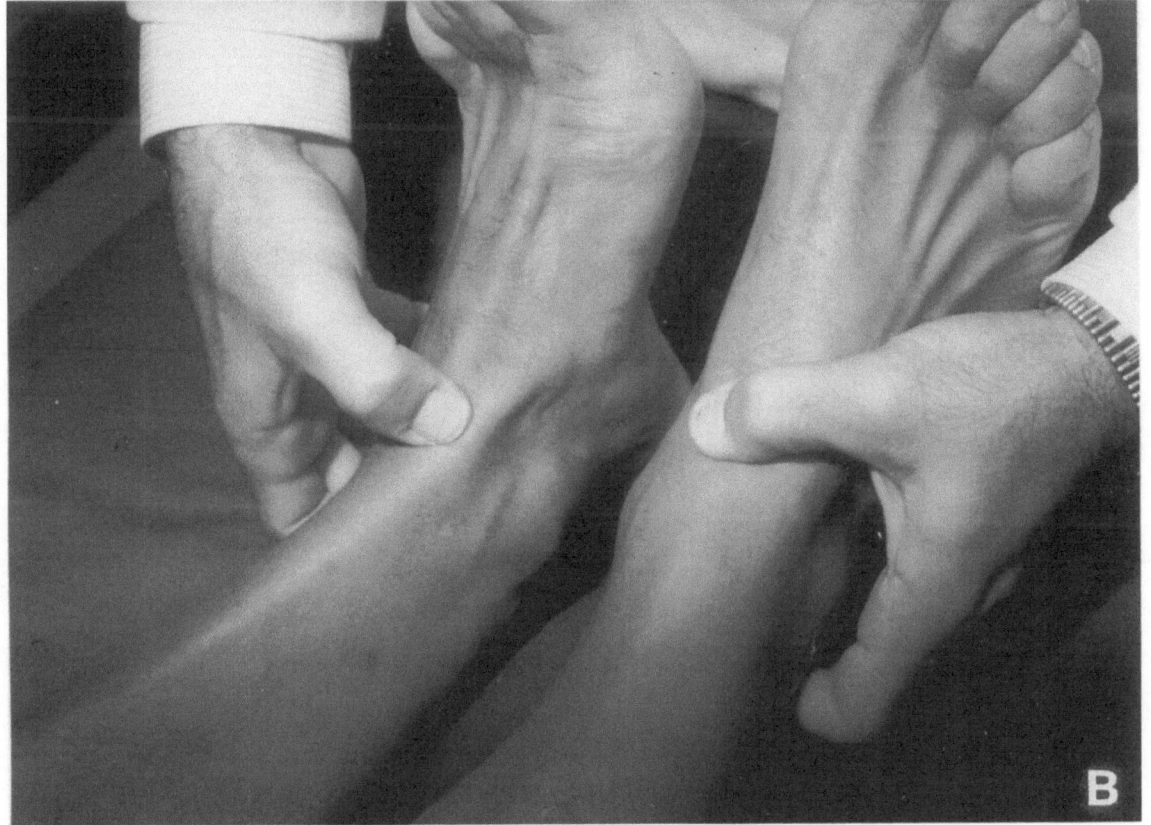

Hyposthenia of the extensor hallucis brevis (A) indicates pathology of the root at L_5, and thus disc pathology between L_4 and L_5.

The same goes for deficit of the extensor digitorum communis.

Hypovalidity, or the absence of the Achilles reflex (B) reveals pathology of the nerve root at S_1, and, thus, disc pathology between L_5 and S_1.

The same may be said for deficit of the mid-plantar reflex.

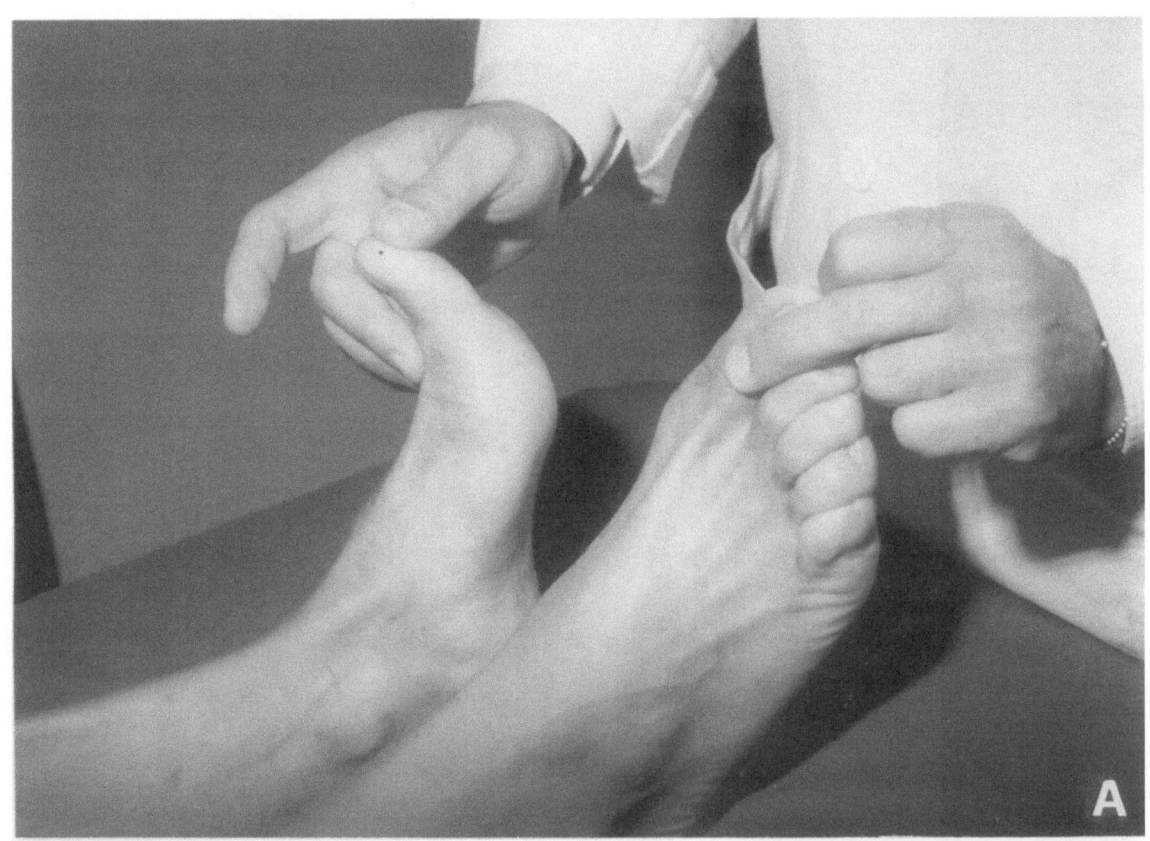

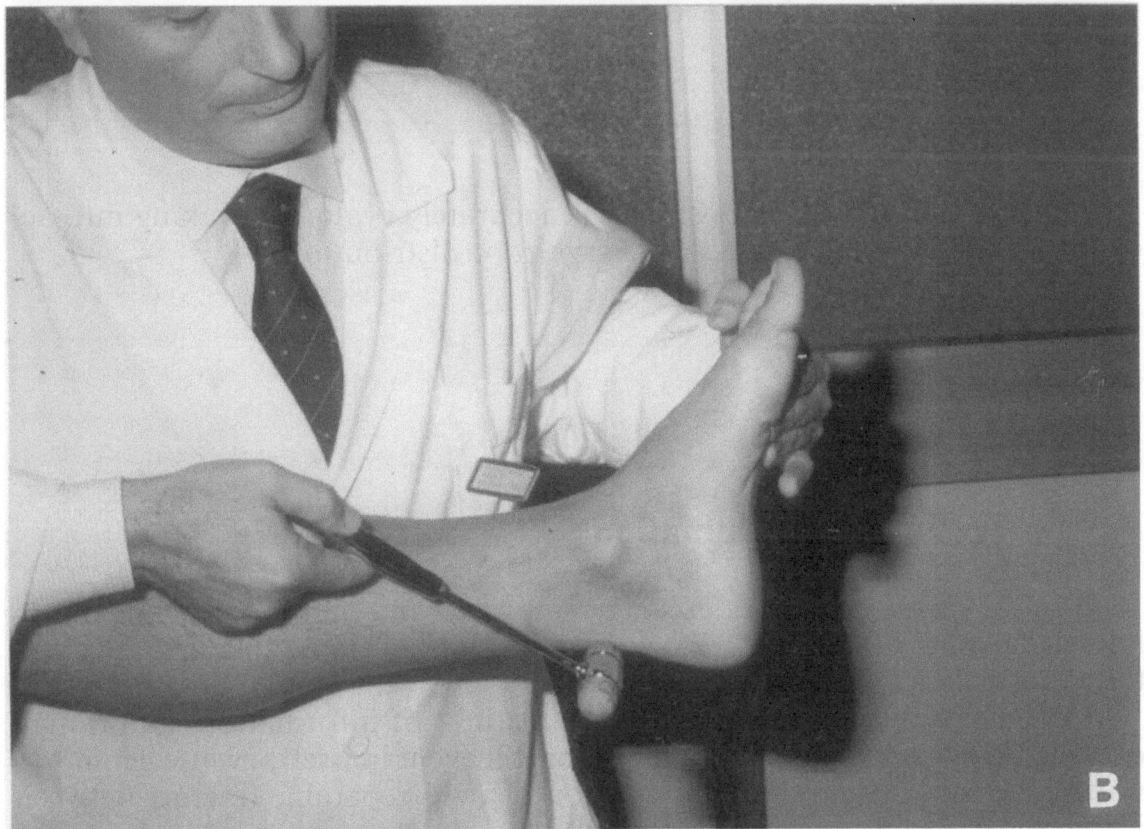

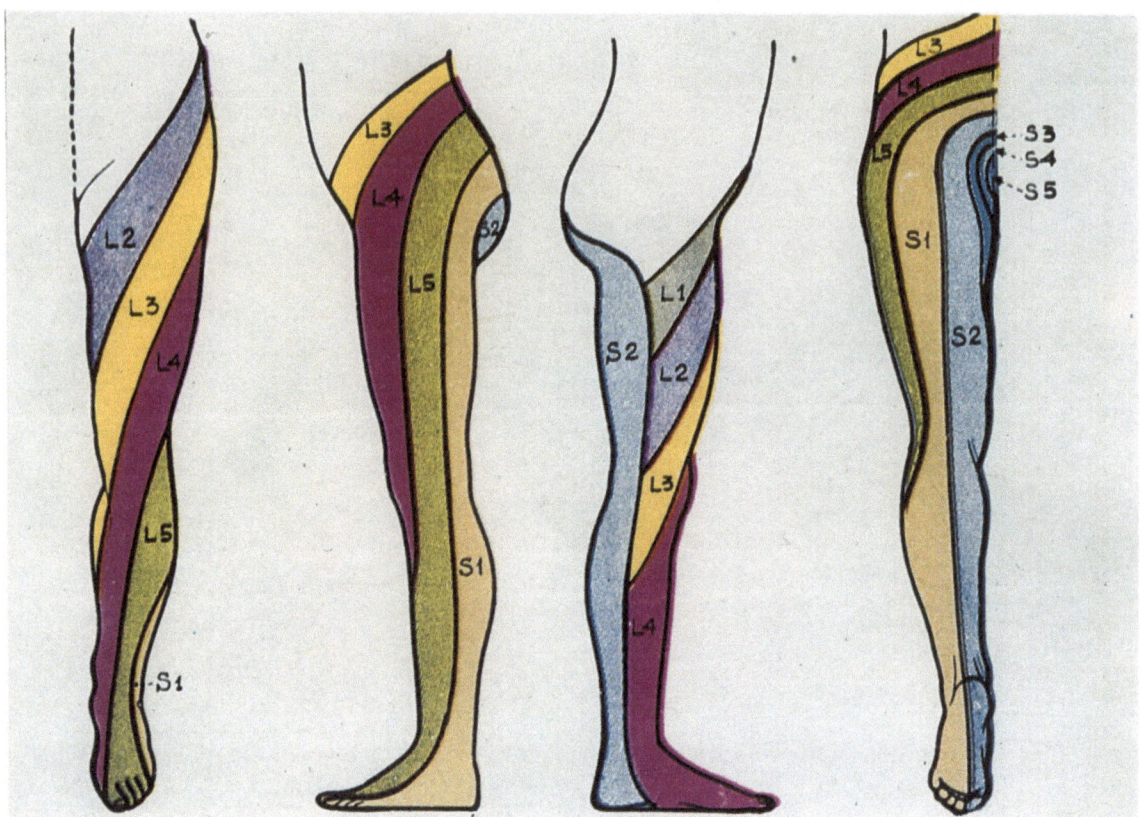

Disorder in superficial sensitivity is accurately evaluated, taking into account the dermatomeric areas of nerve root distribution.

Psychoalgesimetric examination

Acute pain may be considered a «symptom» and thus a «principle of acknowledgement» (Melzack, 1965) of a pathological state, an alarm reaction to actual deficit.

Chronic pain does not possess these features of information, and it may often itself become «disease», a pathological event in itself, even when it has no organic substratum, the manifestation of an «irreparable fracture between being and knowing» (Bocchi, 1980).

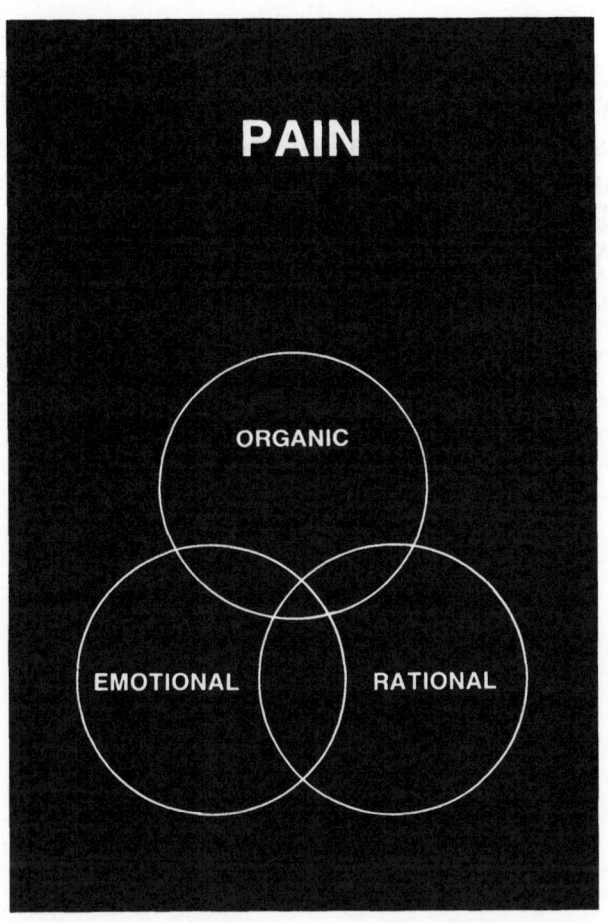

Psychological factors (motivational, affective, cognitive, emotional, perceptive, ethnic, environmental, etc.) play different roles in the procedures with which:

1) the experience of pain is perceived, intensifying or predicting the transmission of nociceptive afferences to the brain;

2) it is possible to determine the reactive behavior to these experiences (reactions of «having been used»: mimicking, verbalization, etc.).

Psychological evaluation*

The choice of this test is based on several considerations: the amount of time required for use, the simplicity and comprehensibility of the questions, whether or not there is a sufficient psychological profile, which is then delineated for routine therapeutic needs.

1) Taylor anxiety questionnaire
2) Rockliff self-rating questionnaire for depression (SRQ-D)
3) Crown and Crisp (MHQ) self-rating questionnaire for psychoneurotic patients.

* See Appendix, p. 125

Algesimetric classification systems

In order to evaluate the long-term results of therapy, these tests are flanked by algesimetric classification systems which, among all of those proposed by various authors, we felt to be the most reliable, and the easiest to apply:
1) Verbal analogue for pain (VRS-Verbal Rating Scale) (A)
2) Visual analogue for pain (VAS-Visual Analogue Scale) (B)
3) Achromatic pain scale (series of Luescher grays) (C)

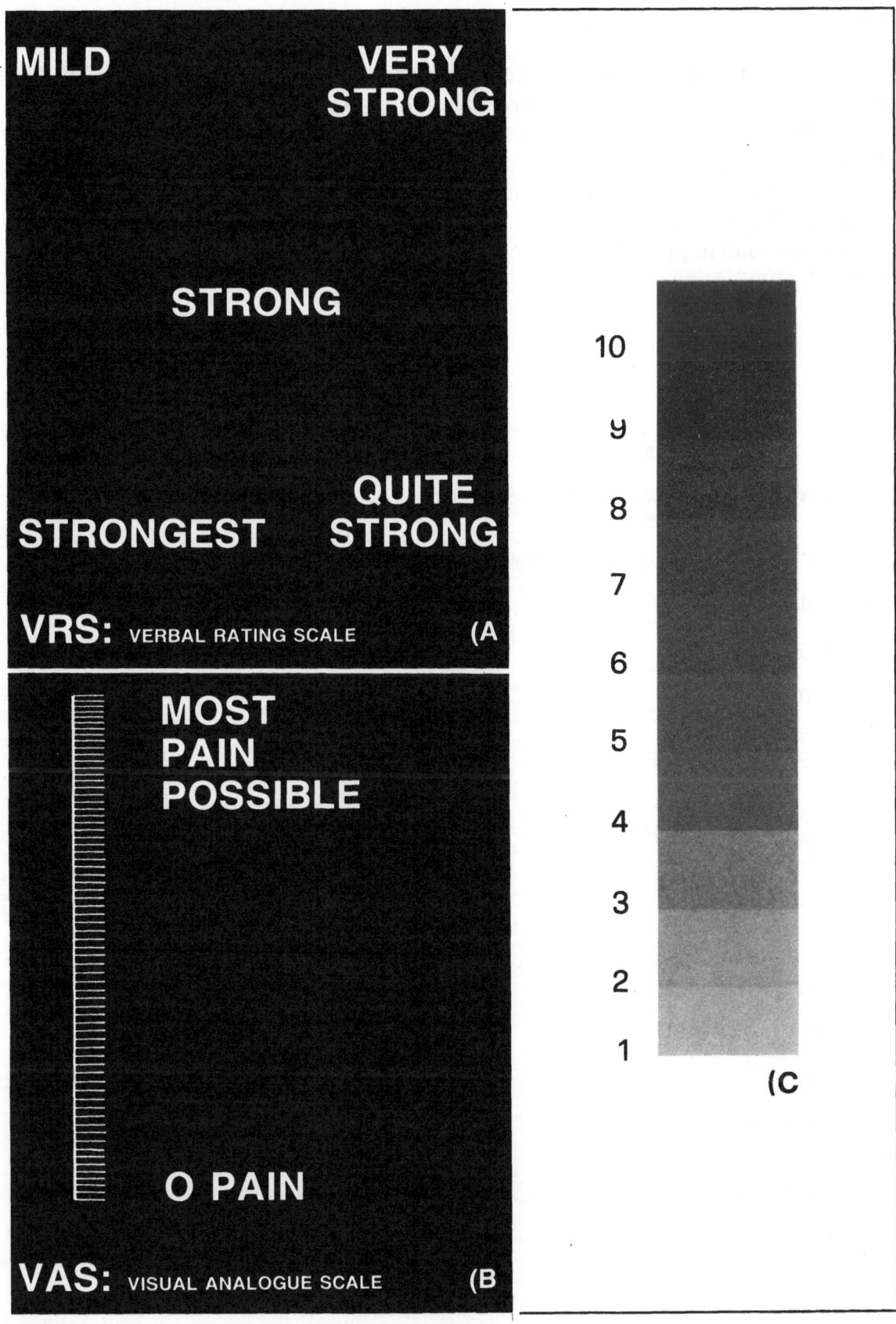

MILD   VERY STRONG

STRONG

STRONGEST   QUITE STRONG

VRS: VERBAL RATING SCALE   (A

MOST PAIN POSSIBLE

O PAIN

VAS: VISUAL ANALOGUE SCALE   (B

10
9
8
7
6
5
4
3
2
1

(C

Psychoalgesimetric record

The results of these evaluations are then summarized in the *Individual psychoalgesimetric record*, where the values obtained are recorded.

A clinical and psychological evaluation allowed us to classify three groups of algic patients:

1) patients with predominantly somatic pain;

2) patients with predominantly psychogenic pain;

3) psychiatric patients (severe depression, hysteria, other psychiatric disorders).

PSYCHOALGESIMETRIC RECORD

Name .... Surname .... Age .... Sex ....

Clinical record n. .... Date of evaluation .... Diagnosis....................

PSYCHOLOGICAL EVALUATION		Score
Taylor		....
SRQ-D		....
MHQ	Anxiety	....
	Phobias	....
	Obsessions	....
	Somatic disorders	....
	Depression	....
	Hysteria	....

ALGESIMETRIC EVALUATION	
VRS	....
VAS	....
Achromatic	....

COMMENTS ....

....

The examiner

Let us now try to classify the possible typologies of patients characterized by a strong pain component.

Type A, free of important psychological problems, should be able to be successfully treated by medical therapy.

Type B, although free of important psychological problems, is a subject who has difficulty tolerating the role of the patient and, if hospitalized, he or she manifests anxiety and depression. These are usually very active persons, who see the state of illness as a sort of handicap; usually, however, once the noxa pathogena has been removed, psychological problems regress.

Type C does have psychological problems, but he or she is able to manage a good relationship with himself and with others, although this patient must make a considerable psychological effort to do so. As the disease begins, the patient's psychological problems are added to his organic ones, so that the symptom of pain may last even after the disease itself has been successfully treated.

Type D combines the negative effects of his or her organic and psychological discomfort. The perception of pain is exaggerated and it may last even after the organic aspect of the problem has been successfully treated.

Type	Organic state	Psychological state	Risk level
A	Severe organic problem	No important psychological problem	None or mild
B	Severe organic problem	Depression and anxiety caused by disease. No previous signs of psychological discomfort	Low
C	Severe organic problem	Latent psychological problems triggered by disease	Average to high
D	Severe organic problem	Psychological problems prior to disease	High
E	Average to mild organic problem	Mild psychological problems	Average
F	Average to mild organic problem	Psychological problems prior to disease	High
G	Mild to non-existent organic problem	Severe neurosis or psychosis	High

Type E tends to start up a feed-back type of relationship between what is psychological and what is organic, with reciprocal influence: pain and state of depression are exalted, producing a vicious cycle. In cases such as these the physician always needs the help of a psychologist.

Type F in practice acts like type D: the organic disorder is the basis on which psychosomatic construction is based. Pain is amplified and nearly certainly destined to last after surgery.

Type G is characterized by severe neurosis or psychosis; consequently, the surgeon is not needed, rather, the help of a psychiatrist and a psychotherapist is.

Diagnostic examinations

B. Paschero

General information

Percutaneous discectomy according to the Onik method requires an accurate instrumental evaluation of the patients to be treated by the method.

The tools available guaranteeing an accurate selection of the patients are currently:
— Computerized Tomography
— Myeloradiculography
— Magnetic Resonance Tomography.

None of these examinations, however, are capable of correctly defining the state of contained herniation, and, thus, indicating use of a percutaneous discectomy; these examinations instead easily provide criteria for exclusion.

Moreover, the amount of time between ascertainment and surgery must be taken into account: during this period of time, a specific anatomic and pathological situation may change, and a disc protrusion, defined «contained», may at surgery become an actual «extruded» herniation. For these reasons, we consider intraoperative discography to be essential in selecting patients to be submitted to discectomy.

This affirmation is further proven by our experience.

When we first began to use the Onik method, all of the patients were chosen based on the data provided by computerized tomography, myeloradiculography, magnetic resonance tomography. In this first group, intraoperative discography revealed a picture of extruded hernia in 10% of the cases.

The clearly defined representations of anatomic and antomopathological reality provided by third generation computerized tomography led us to perform percutaneous discectomy in patients for whom significant images of contained disc hernia were revealed by computerized tomography. In this second group, intraoperative discography again showed a picture of extruded disc herniation in 10% of the cases.

This agreement in diagnostic error between the two groups convinced us that computerized tomography is sufficient for a first selection of patients to be submitted to percutaneous discectomy, leaving the final verdict up to intraoperative discography.

This takes nothing away from the value of the other instrumental methods in the diagnosis of this pathology of the intervertebral disc. In our opinion, however, other tests must be restricted to those cases in which diagnosis is doubtful, and which computerized tomography would not be able to solve, and in which it would be hazardous to perform discography.

Let us recall that to be effective any ascertainment must be carried out according to the rules, using any technical device that may help to reveal any disc pathology, and to distinguish it from other pathologies, thus avoiding the risk of the data degrading.

Computerized tomography

In evaluating a computerized tomographic examination the scout-view is important (A), a simil-radiographic image which should occur at the onset of the series of tomograms. Three broken lines appear, corresponding to the graphic representation of the series of tomograms carried out, and which indicate the inclination of the gantry. These lines must be parallel to the disc space to be studied.

With this orientation the image marked by an X corresponds to a level which is equidistant from the somatic plates (B). In this case there is right paramedian disc protrusion at this level.

However, it is important to always carry out a tomogram 3 mm above (X + 3) and 3 mm below (X - 3) the level, to reveal the presence of any protruded disc material which may have ascended cranially (C) or descended caudally (D).

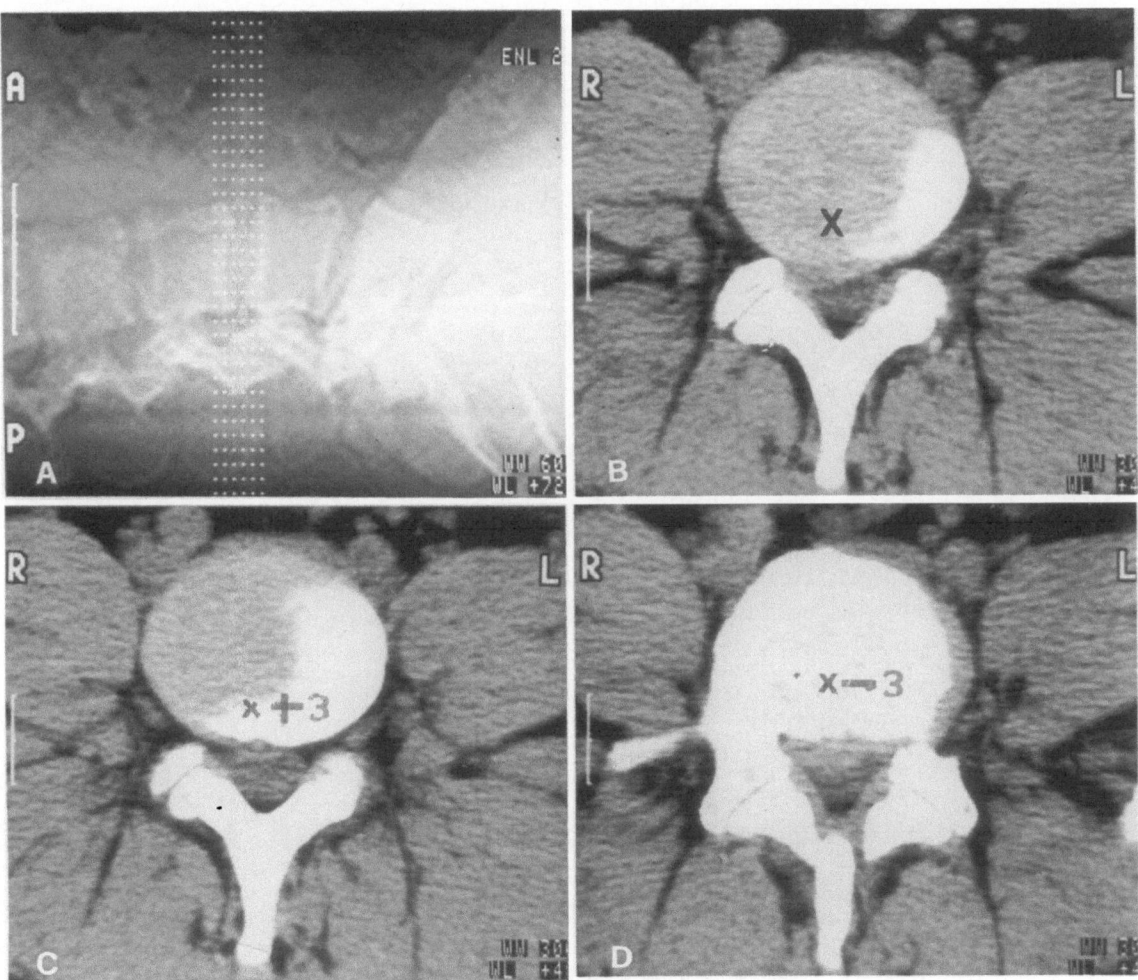

A, B) The tomographic image may be processed in such a way as to show an isodensity between the tissue present in the disc space and any protruded tissue, thus ascertaining its identity. In this case of right paramedian disc herniation at L_4-L_5, image intensifier is used to make points with the same gray intensity show up more and shine, which, for instance, makes it possible to distinguish between disc tissue and non-disc tissue.

Series of four axial tomograms of disc herniations which are apparently contained: right paramedian disc herniation at L_5-S_1 (C), right paramedian disc herniation at L_5-S_1 (D), right lateral disc herniation at L_4-L_5 (E), left lateral disc herniation at L_4-L_5 (F). The latter are generally defined by radiologists to be foraminal. In truth, they correspond to a more lateral protrusion of the disc, which reduces the caliber of the conjugate foramen.

Common to all four of the images are the rounded borders of the disc protrusion: a supposition of contained hernia.

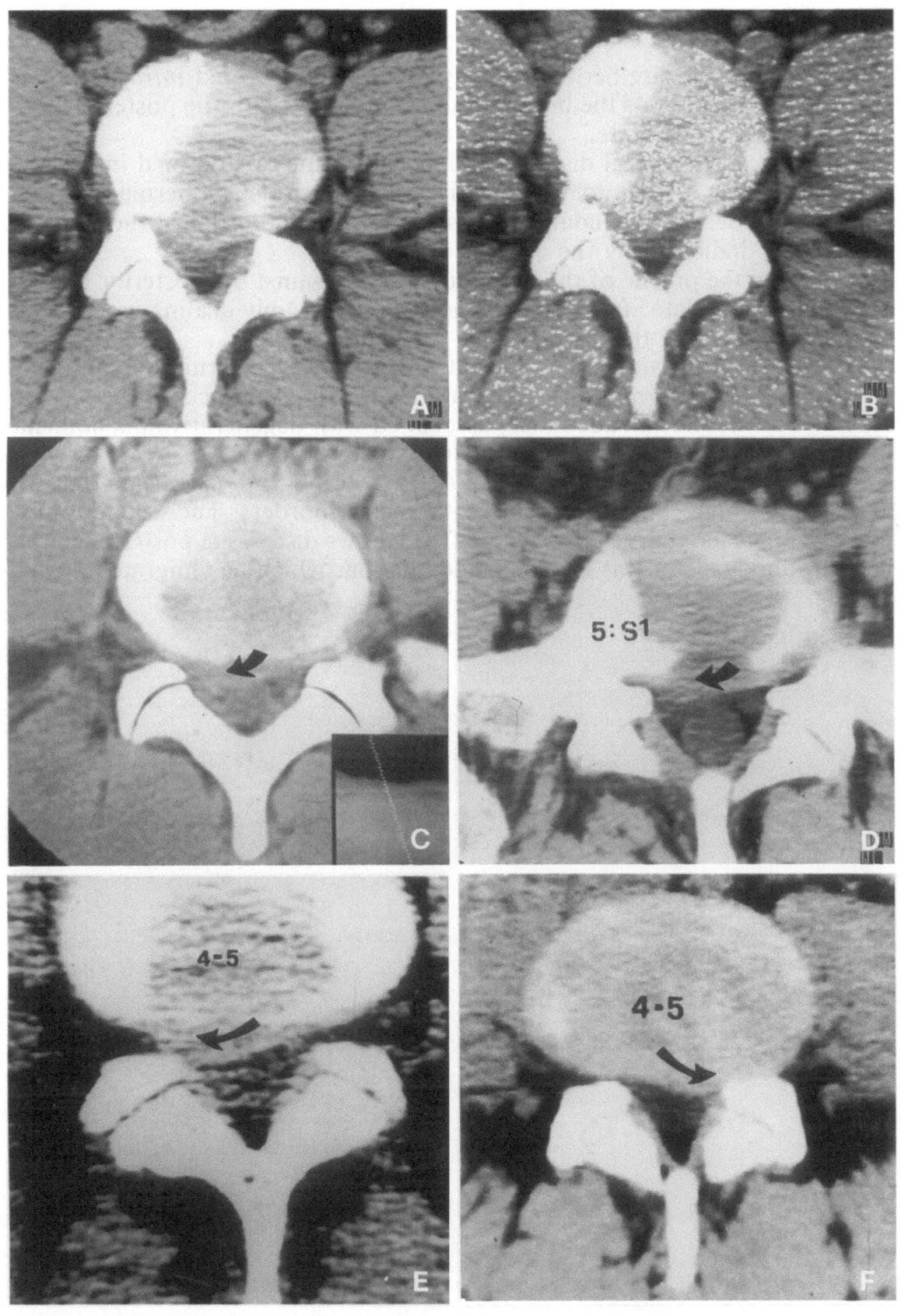

Criteria for exclusion

A) CT scan of disc herniation may really be considered *intraforaminal* as the medial profile of the hernia is at a *right angle* with the posterior border of the vertebral plate.

B) CT scan of lateral disc herniation, which may be defined intraforaminal according to radiological criteria. Probably, this is a hernia which is already extruded, as it caudally surpasses the skeletal border of the somatic plate of L_4, indicated by the arrow.

C) When the profile of the hernia comes up against the posterior border of the vertebral plate at an *acute angle*, we are probably dealing with an extruded hernia, as in this case of disc herniation at L_5-S_1.

D) CT scan of paramedian and intraforaminal disc herniation with **calcification**. This is a symptom of a pathology which is not recent. The picture indicates a veterate extruded disc, associated with degenerative phenomena in the somatic plate, as well (images of erosion).

E, F) Disc herniation at L_4-L_5. In the first tomogram it appears that we are dealing with a contained hernia with unclear borders. The second tomogram, 3 mm caudal in relation to the first, shows disc tissue posterior to the vertebral body at L_5; this is an extruded hernia, which has migrated downwards.

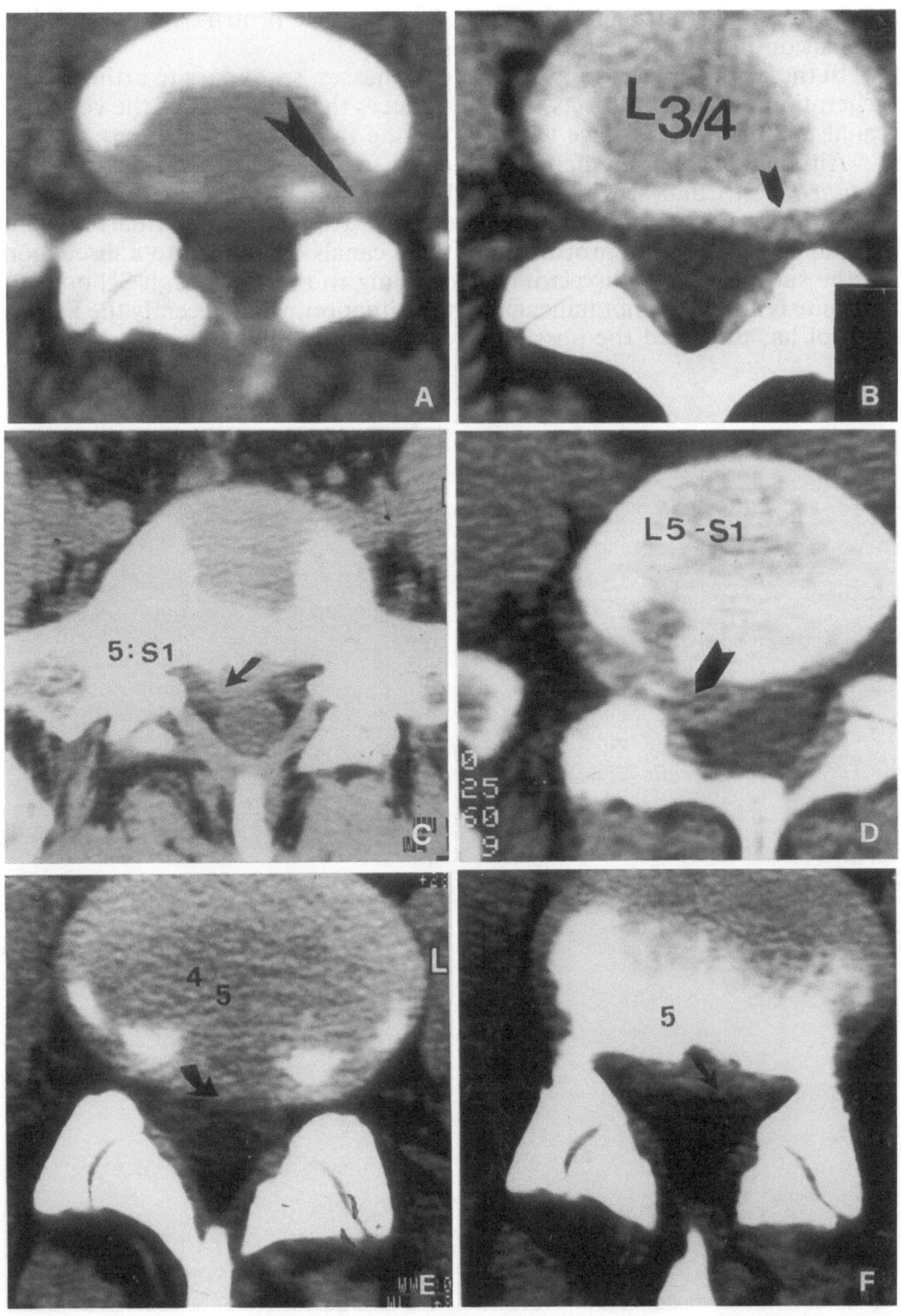

Traditional contraindications are: massive disc protrusion (A) and disc protrusion in narrow arthrosic canals (B).

In these cases hypertrophy of the joint masses, secondary to arthrosis degeneration of the joint facets, further reduces the diameters of the vertebral canal and annuls the space reserved for the radicular connection.

Although discectomy may be indicated for disc protrusions in a narrow *non-arthrosic* canal, it would clearly be useless in a narrow *arthrosic* canal.

C, D, E, F) Tomograms at several levels, from L_3 to L_5 of narrow congenital canal. Any disc protrusion in these canals could lead to a discussion of the suitability of a discectomy. According to the Pittsburgh School discectomy is absolutely not indicated in this situation, while recently the French School has discussed the possibility of using just this method.

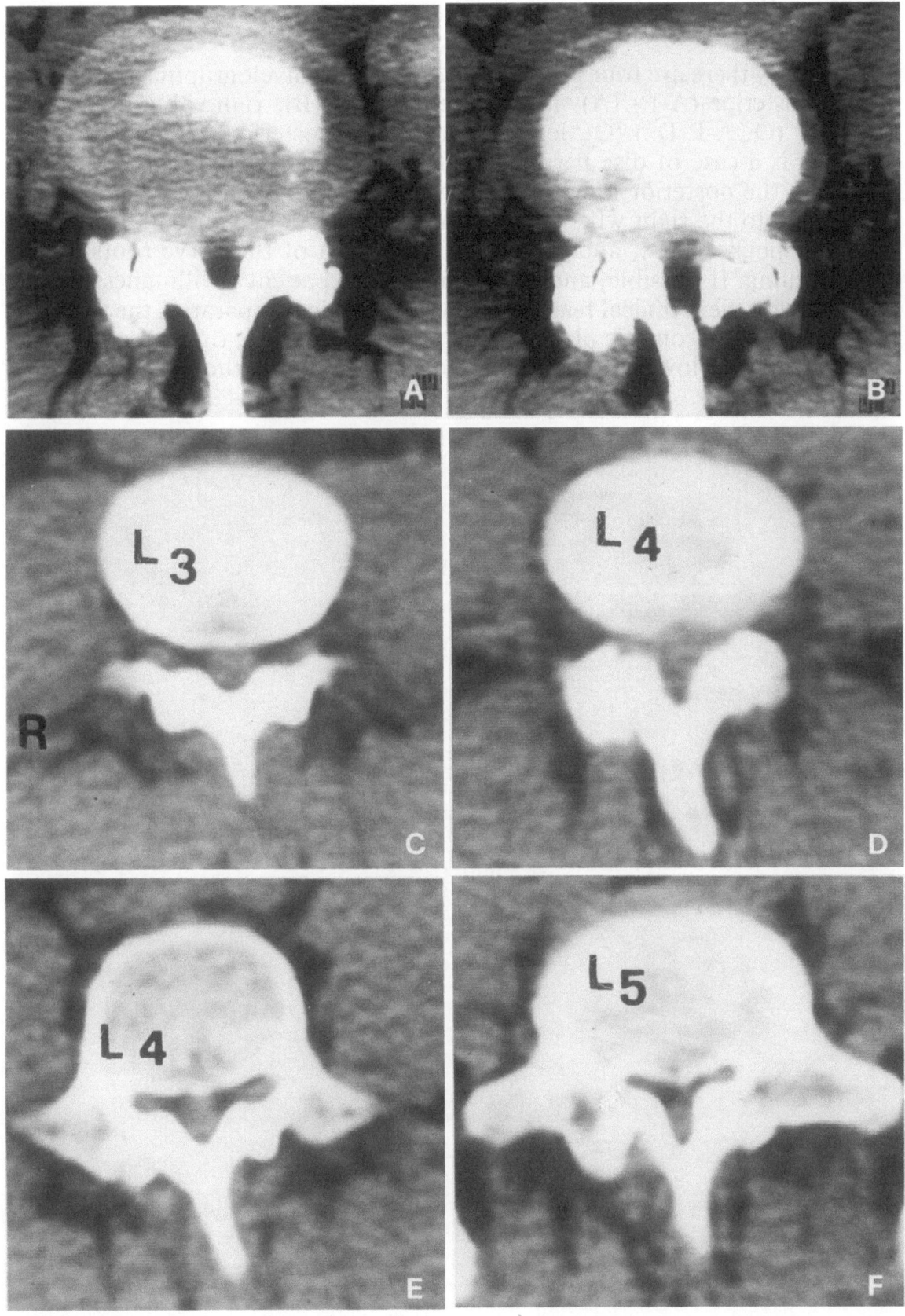

Myeloradiculography

Basically there are four projections essential to myelographic evaluation: antero-posterior (A-P) (A), latero-lateral (L-L) (B), right oblique antero-posterior (O. A-P Dx) (C), left oblique antero-posterior (O. A-P Sn) (D).

This is a case of disc herniation at L_4-L_5 which is apparently still contained by the posterior longitudinal ligament, and which is prevalently extrinsecated to the right where it determines the complete amputation of the radicular pocket at L_5, and stringing phenomena of the nerve roots of the cauda equina. If possible, and depending on the patient's willingness to collaborate with the technical features of the radiological apparatus, the ray must be parallel to the somatic plates of the pathological disc, thus obtaining images which best allow for an evaluation of the anatomopathological situation.

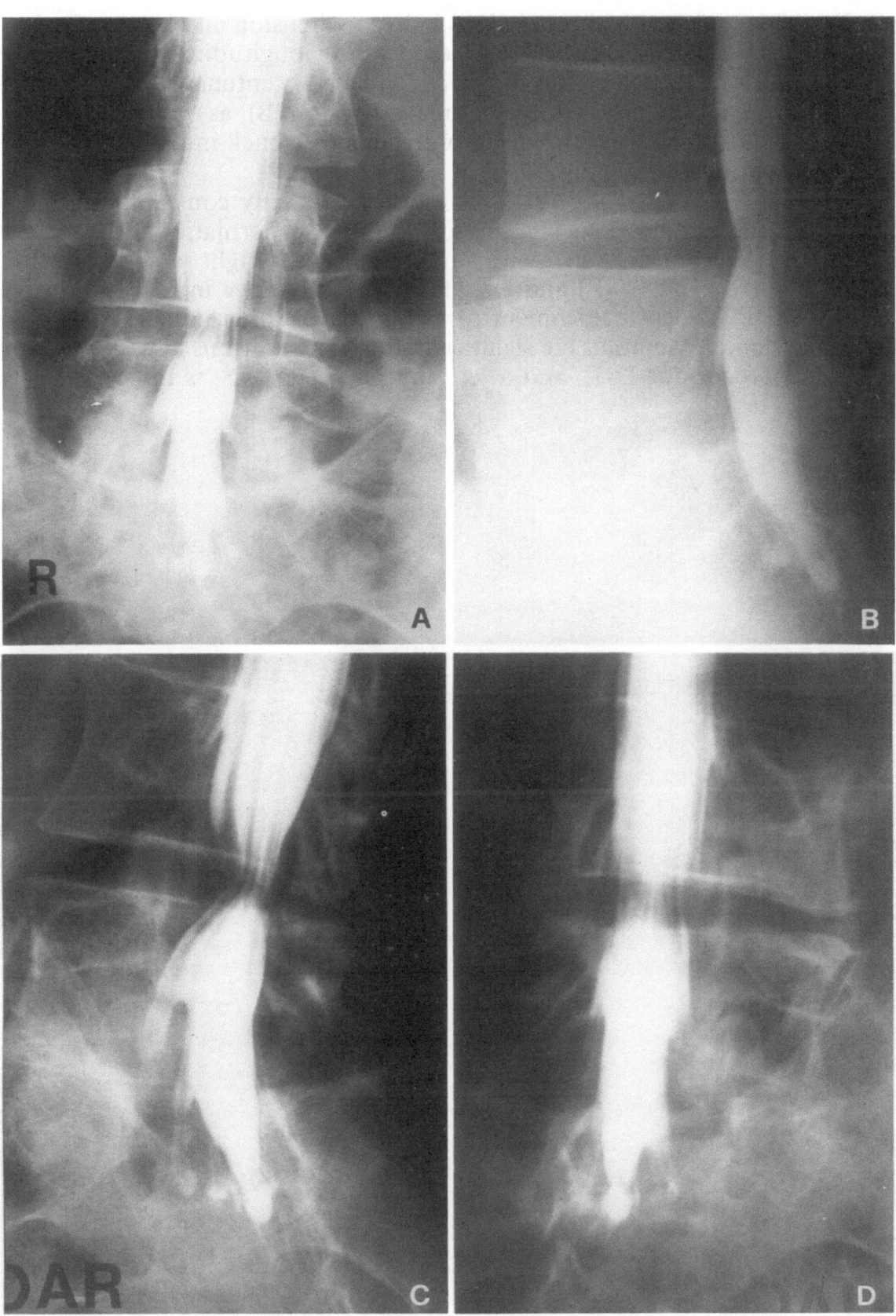

Dynamic or functional projections in hyperextension and hyperreflexion may inform us on the integrity of the posterior longitudinal ligament.

In this case, the impression on the dural sac is accentuated with hyperextension (A), and is clearly reduced with hyperflexion (B), as the whole posterior longitudinal ligament pushes the protruded disc back into its site. These images, as well, must be obtained in orthostatism.

Disk impressions at several levels do not generally contraindicate percutaneous discectomy. This is a case of double disc herniation at L_4-L_5 and L_5-S_1 (C), which is manifested with amputation of the right radicular pocket of the nerve root at L_5 (E) and left at S_1 (F). The image in L-L projection (D) shows no evident detachment of the posterior longitudinal ligament.

If the clinical symptoms are significant, dual percutaneous discectomy with a right approach for L_4-L_5 and a left approach for L_5-S_1 is indicated.

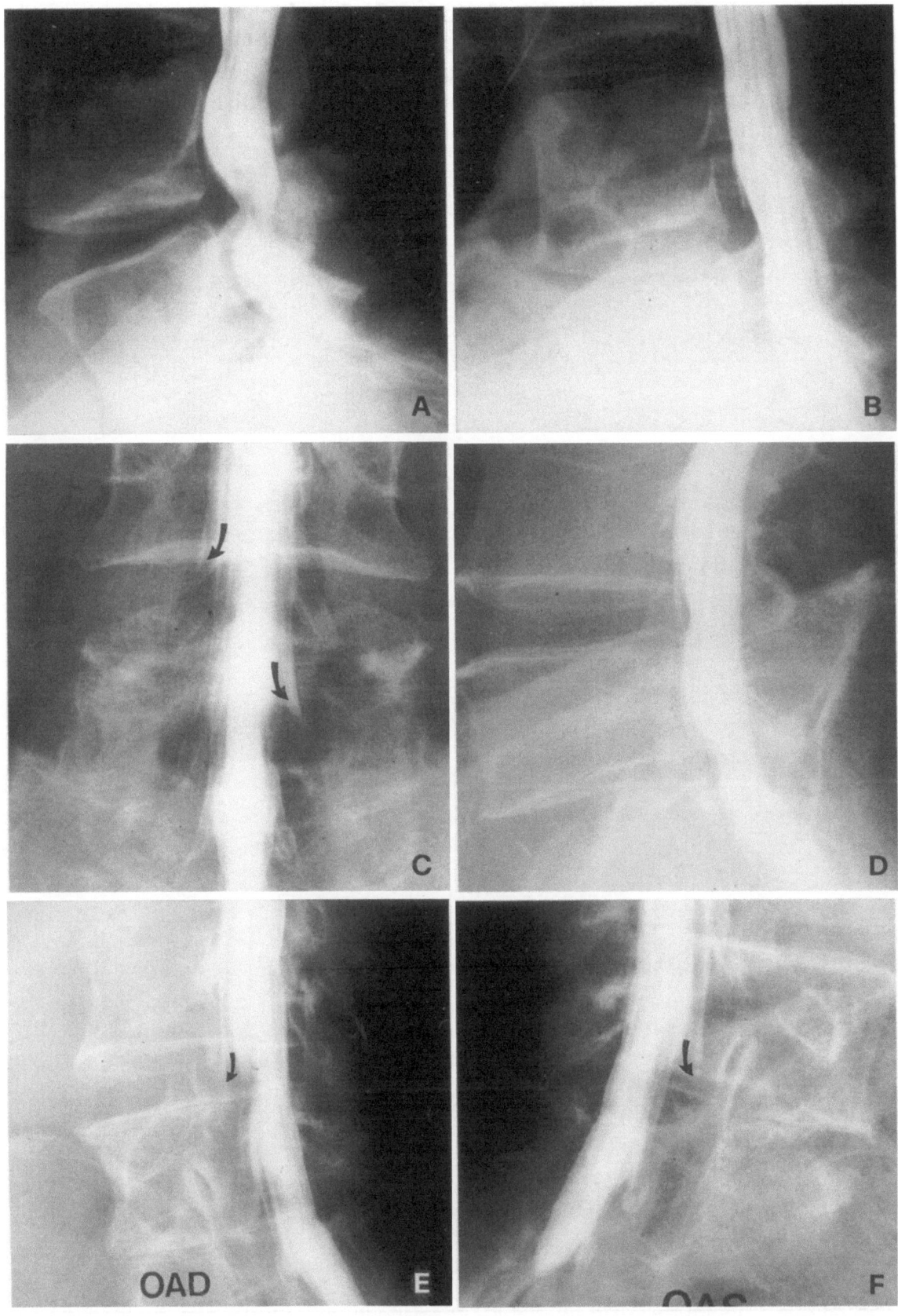

A, B, C, D) Median disc herniation at L_4-L_5 which determines a nearly symmetrical compression of the radicular pockets of L_5. The **symmetry** of the compression may be considered a criterion used to discriminate **contained disc herniation**, as it may lead us to imagine a uniform disc protrusion which with CT scan (E) appears to have rounded borders.

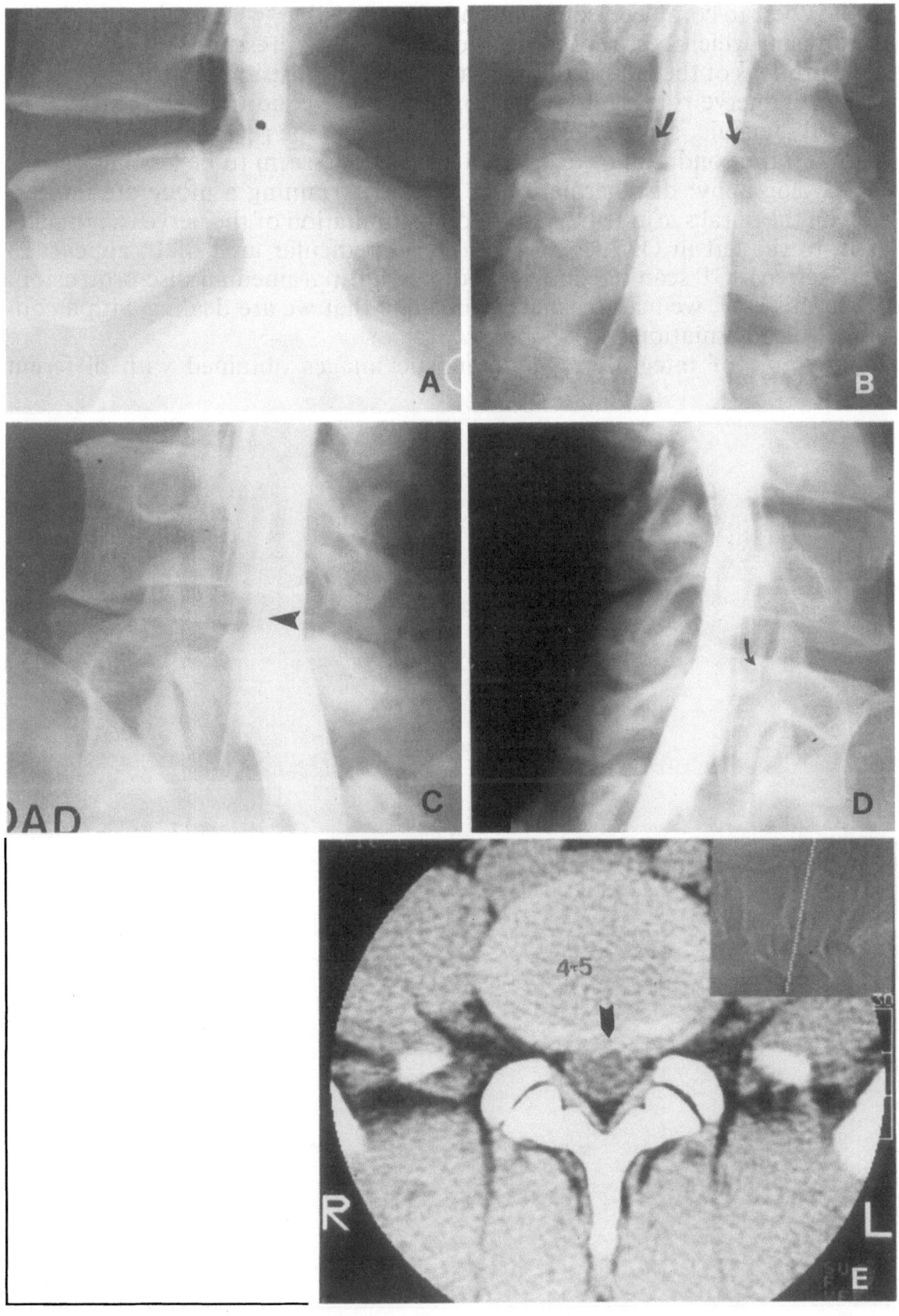

It is best to complete examination, when possible, with projections in **orthostatism**, which best reproduce the state of disc pressure that may determine prolaxis of the anulus fibrosus and thus a protrusion of disc tissue, triggering the nerve root symptomatology. In these conditions, which may be defined dynamic, significant disc protrusion may be revealed, which by CT scan, a static condition of disc hypotension, may seem to be less important.

Myelography: disc herniation at L_4-L_5 determining a moderate impression on the dural sac in L-L (A) and total amputation of the nerve root pocket at L_5 to the left in O. A-P Sn (B) (the subpedicular area of L_5 appears to be deserted). CT scan (C) shows moderate left paramedian disc protrusion.

In this case, we may reasonably imagine that we are dealing with a contained disc herniation.

Example of **integration** of diagnostic images obtained with different methods.

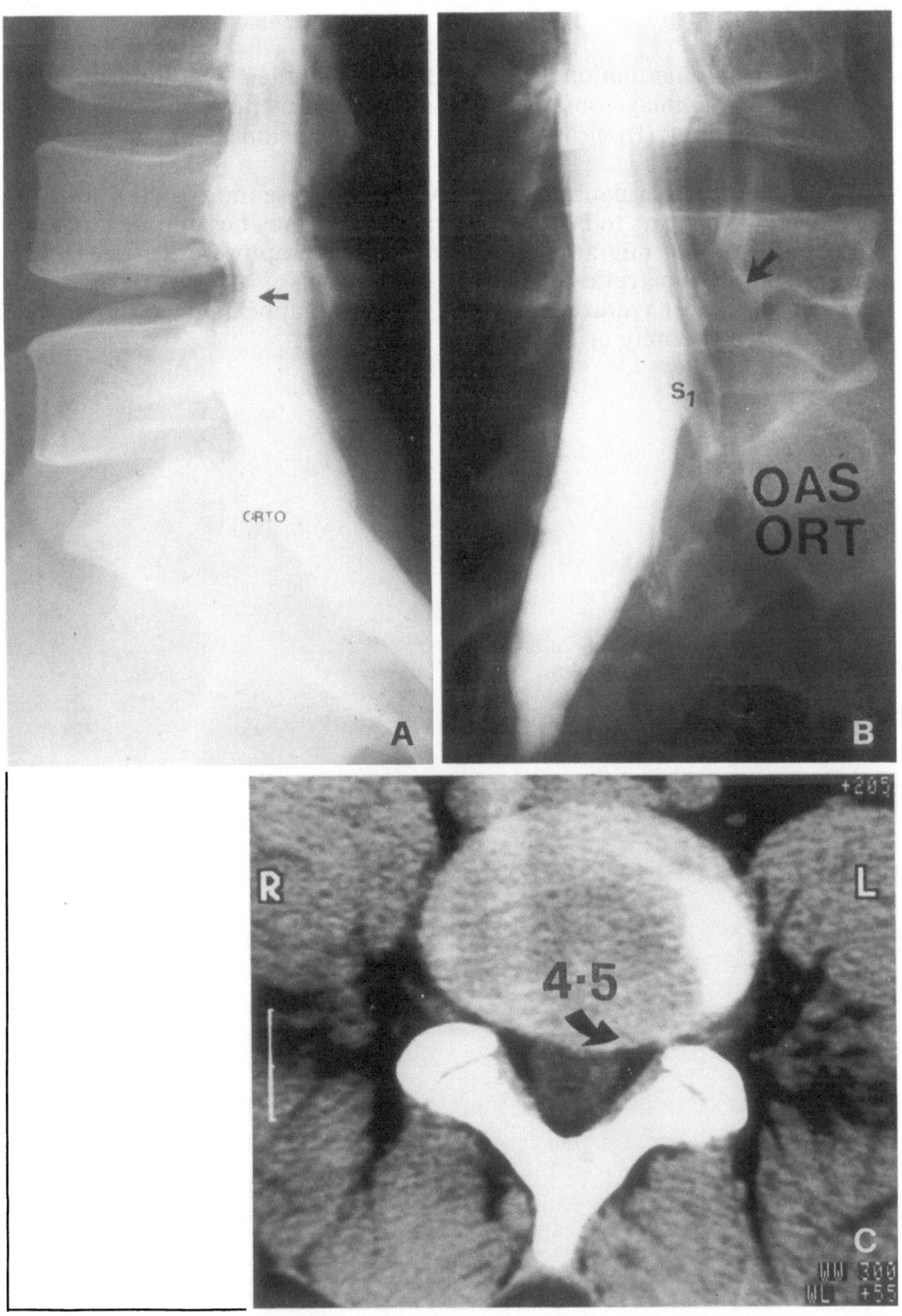

Criteria for exclusion

Extruded disc herniation at L_4-L_5. Observe (A) the correspondence with the myelographic image obtained with nuclear magnetic tomogram. Traditional myelography (B) clearly reveals cranial detachment of the posterior longitudinal ligament.

Protruded disc herniation at L_3-L_4 (C); in this case the posterior longitudinal ligament appears to be detached caudally. It may be supposed that the extruded hernia has migrated downwards. Myelography was carried out in orthostatism in hyperreflexion.

Exclusion: facet syndrome (D): the root at L_5 appears to be amputated by a joint hypertrophy at L_4-L_5.

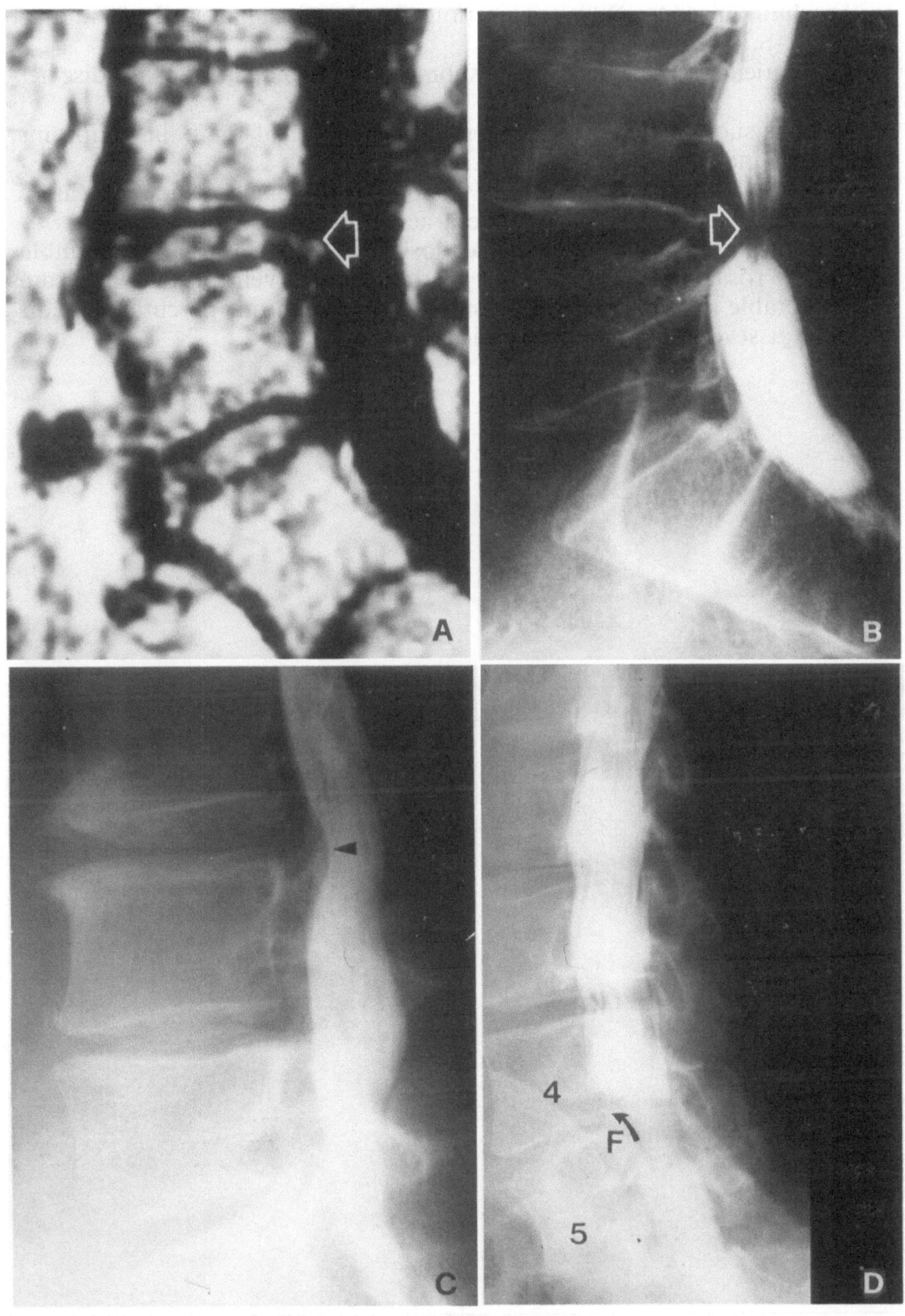

Arachnoiditis: (A, B) two projections for the disc space at L_4-L_5 and for that at L_5-S_1.

This patient had previously been submitted to two operations for disc herniation.

In cases such as these, when there is recurrence of the pain symptoms, there is no indication for percutaneous discectomy.

Observe the rounded borders of the dural cul de sac, which appears to be chainlike, as a result of adhesive arachnoiditis phenomena.

Multiple compression in senile scoliosis: (C, D) the dural sac resembles a string of rosary beads; the turgor of the epidural vein plexuses indicates a considerable amount of compression. In our opinion, percutaneous discectomy at several levels is not indicated.

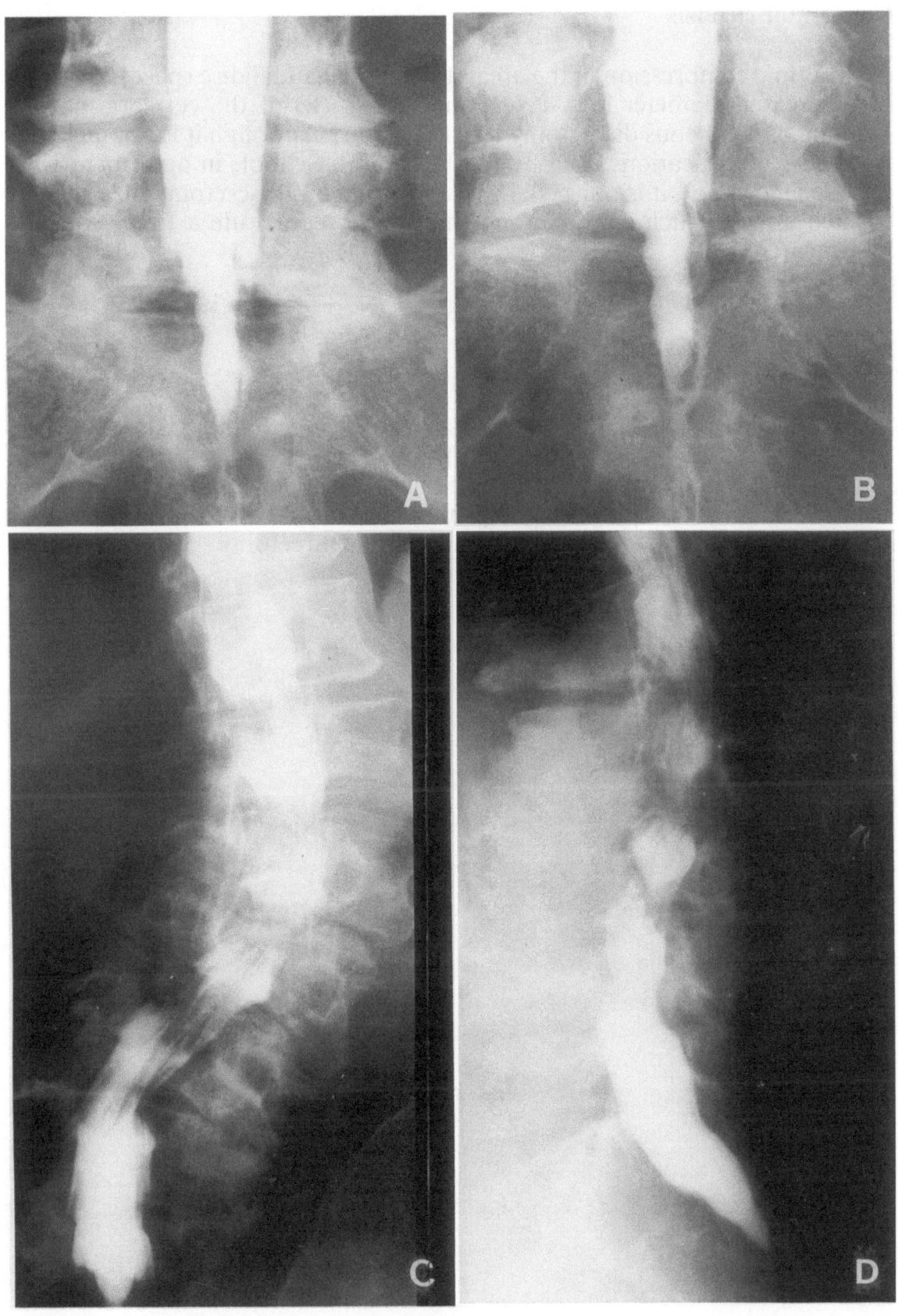

Congenital stenosis

Multiple compression in the area of the more caudal disc spaces. Observe the decreased diameter in A-P (A) and in L-L (B) of the vertebral canal.

Can percutaneous discectomy be carried out? Although it is not included in the list of indications used by the Pittsburgh School, in agreement with the French School, it is our belief that percutaneous discectomy may be performed in cases such as these, and that it may constitute a first choice of treatment.

Arthrosis (C, D)

In addition to the arthrosic impressions (E), myelography shows a large disc herniation at L_5-S_1 to the left (F).

This is a borderline case: could disc herniation benefit from a percutaneous discectomy? Despite the technical difficulties involved, we believe that the best indication is traditional hemilaminoarthrectomy.

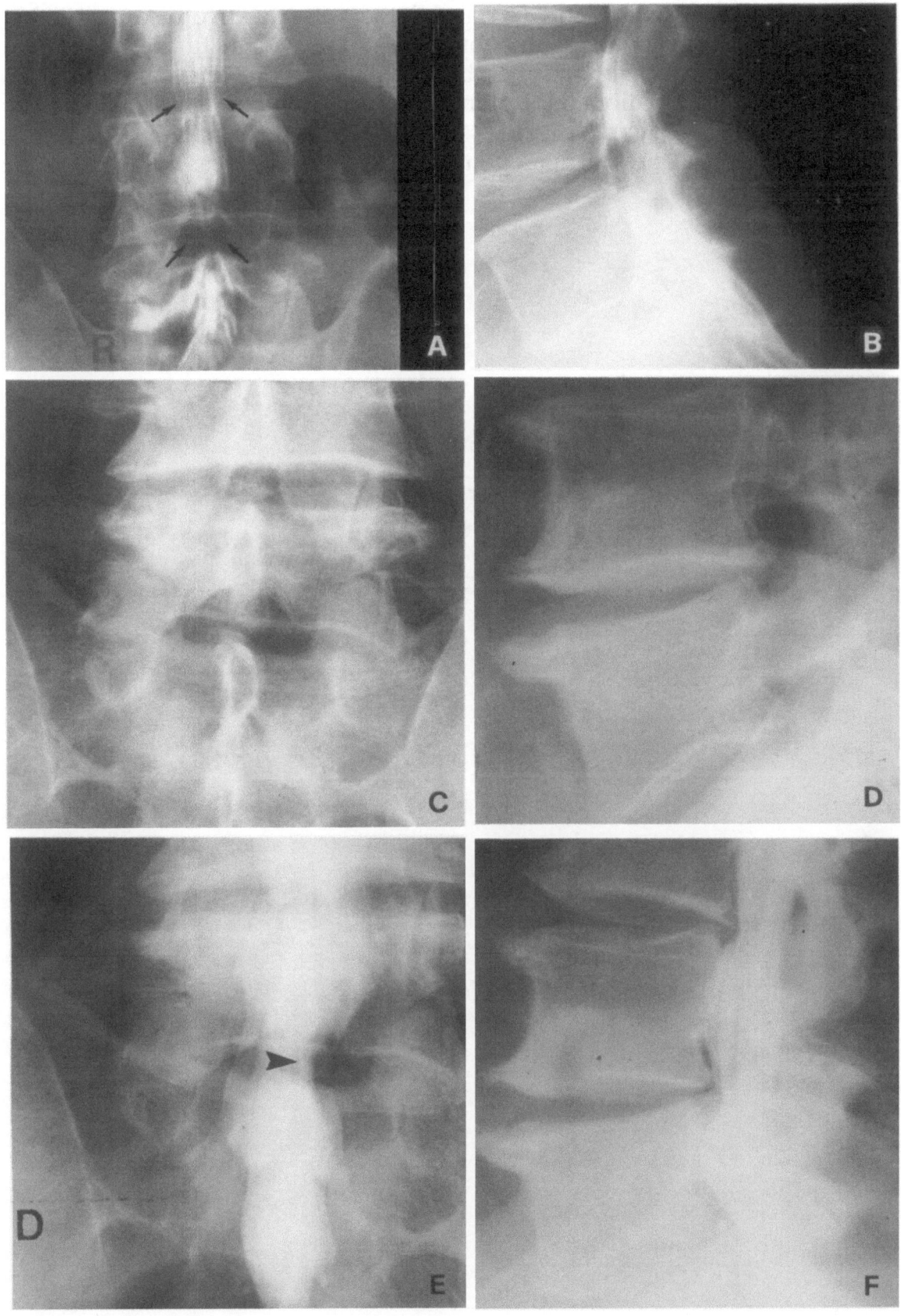

Spondylolisthesis at L_4-L_5 (A) associated with massive disc protrusion (B). Observe in the myelography obtained in A-P (C) the turgor of the vein plexuses, an indication of considerable compression on the dural sac. In L-L projection (D) the radiopaque column appears to be interrupted at the site of the olisthetic vertebra.

Doubtlessly, at present, percutaneous discectomy in cases such as these is contraindicated.

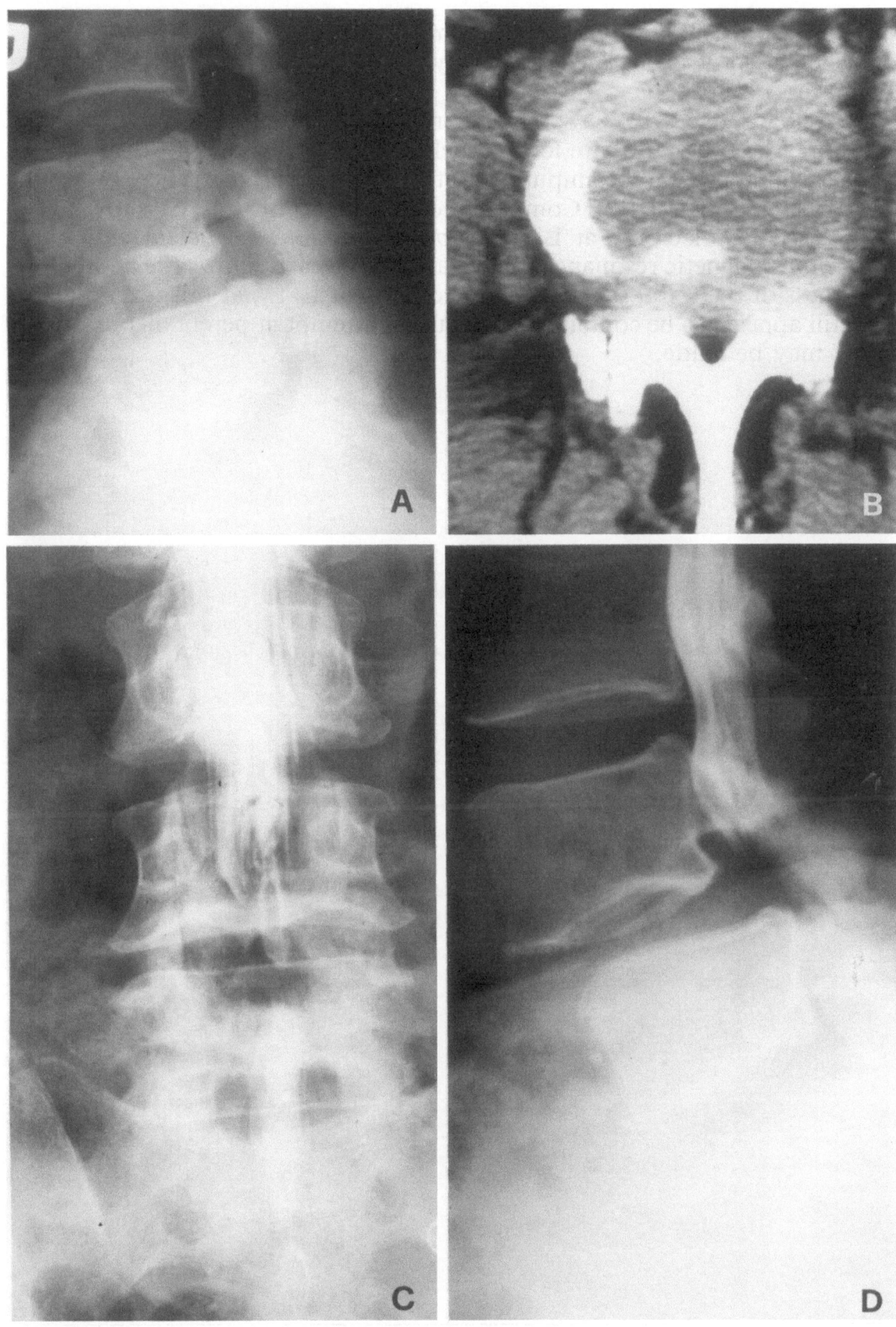

Case of anomaly of the plexus: *pre-fixed plexus*.

The patient was operated previously for disc herniation at L_5-S_1, but obtained no results.

Myelography (A, B, C) reveals the reason for failure: the sac appears to be short; the roots at S_1 are located below the pedicles of L_5; the root at S_1 to the right appears to be amputated, at its anomalous emergence, by a right disc herniation at L_4-L_5. Computerized tomography (D, E) showed the pregressed laminectomy at L_5-S_1: *error related to site due to anatomical variation*. Magnetic resonance tomography (F) clearly shows the anomalous shortness of the dural sac and the discopathy at L_4-L_5; at this level the hernia still appears to be contained and thus an attempt at percutaneous discectomy may be made.

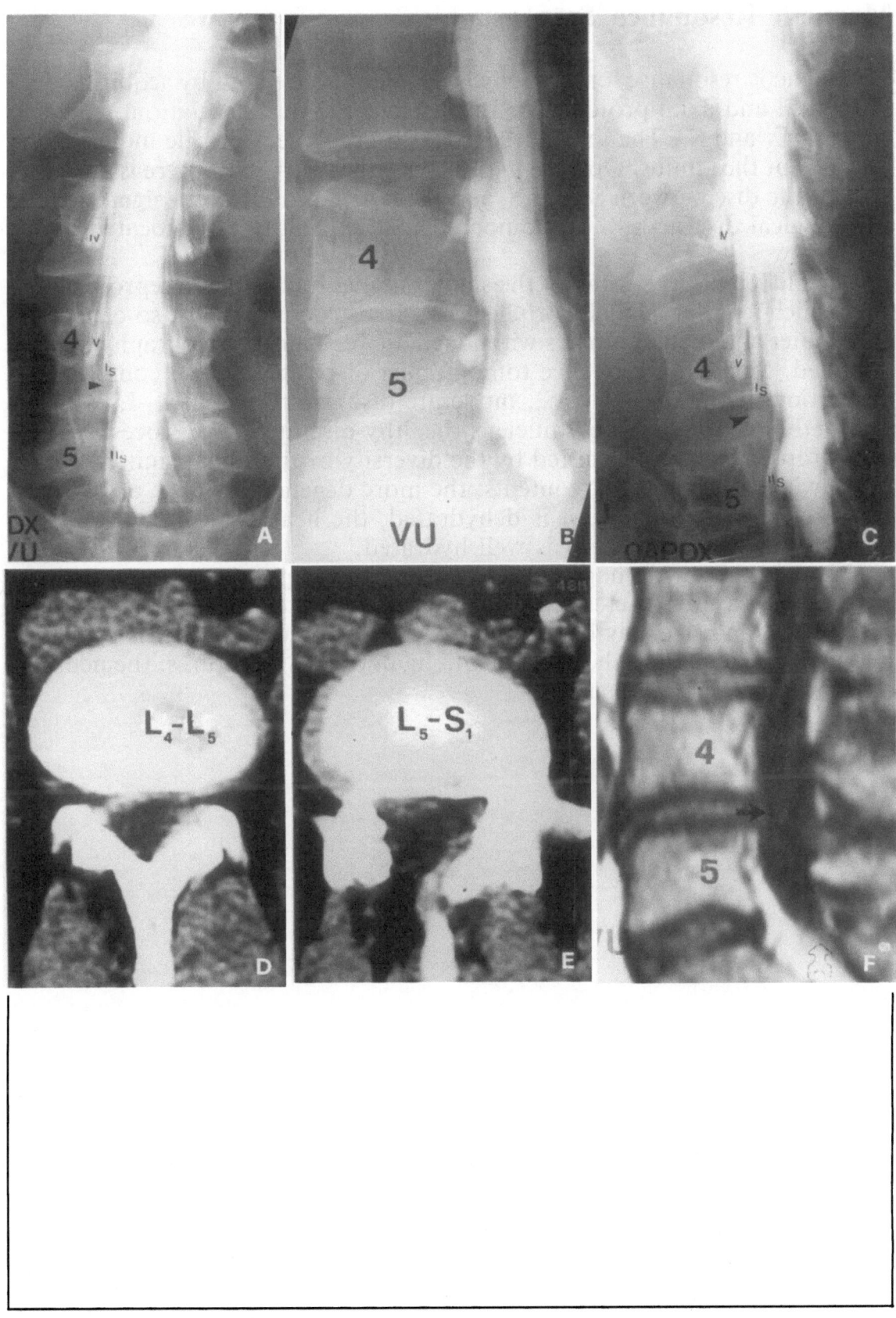

Magnetic Resonance Tomography

Magnetic resonance tomography is routinely carried out by acquiring data in sagittal and axial projections. In this case the disc herniation is located between L_5 and S_1. The axial view (B) with an unclear profile indicates the integrity of the anulus. Observe in the sagittal view (A) that there is a persistence of the disc between S_1 and S_2 and that there is a different signal for the pathological disc at L_5-S_1 as compared to the healthy discs located above and below.

The different processing of the signals makes it possible to reproduce images which iconographically privilege specific structures: thus, so-called discographies and myelographies with magnetic resonance tomography may be obtained. Magnetic resonance tomographic discography (C): complete degeneration of the disc at L_5-S_1, moderate disc protrusion at L_4-L_5 with initial pathology of the pulpy nucleus, healthy disc at L_3-L_4. Processing in a discographic sense is permitted by the diversity of the signal emitted by the tissue with differing water contents: the more degenerated disc, at L_5-S_1 appears to be **dark**, because it is dehydrated, the healthy disc, at L_3-L_4, appears to be **light**, because it is well hydrated.

Myelography with magnetic resonance tomography (D) shows the dural sac, in this case characterized by moderate compression at the L_4-L_5 and L_5-S_1 levels, and size may be determined. A full anatomical view is provided, allowing us to measure the skeletal and ligamentous structures, the neuraxis and the subarachnoid spaces.

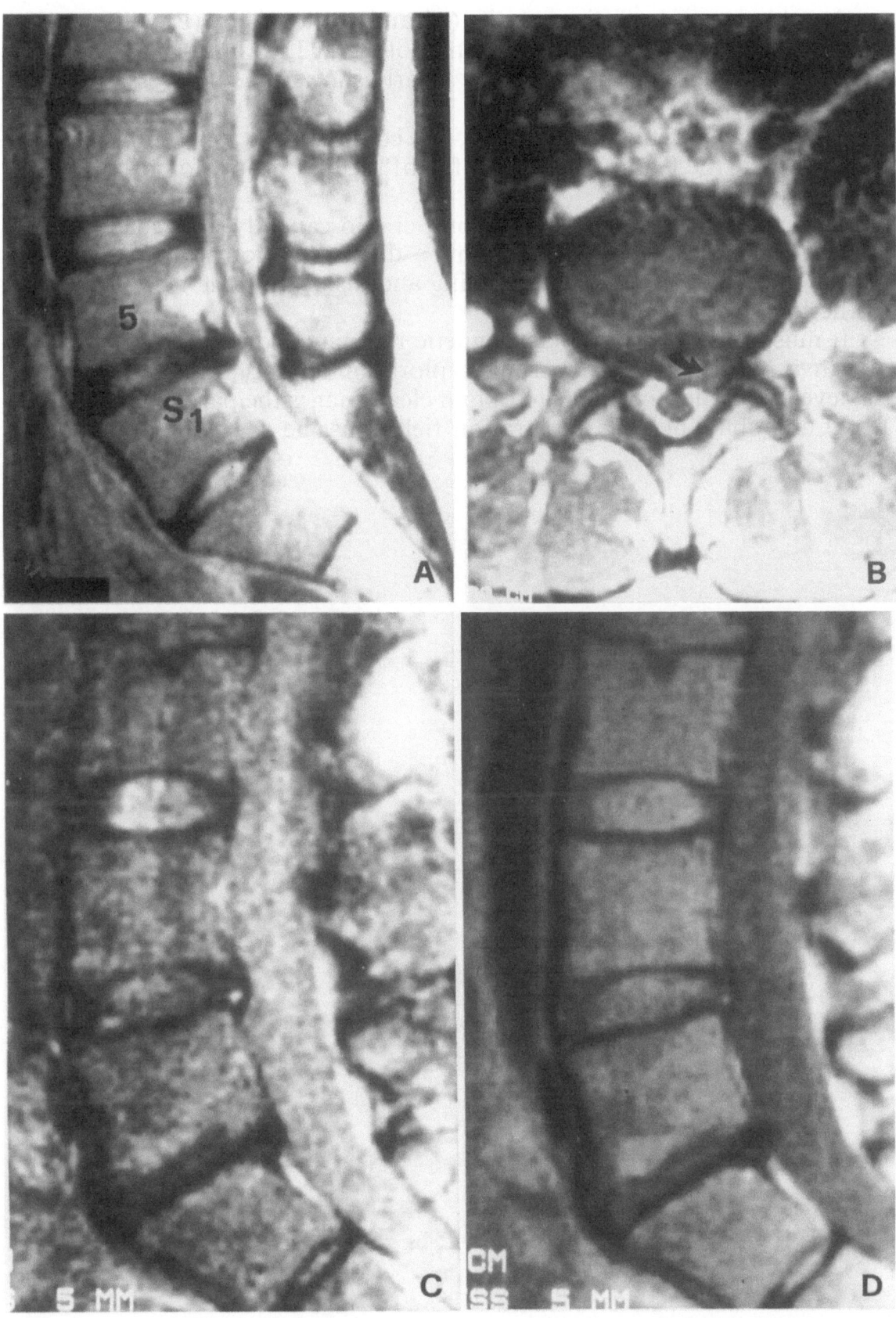

Another example of discography (A) and myelography (B) with magnetic resonance tomography: dual disc pathology at L_4-L_5 and L_5-S_1; magnetic resonance tomography myelography clearly shows the compression on the dural sac at the L_5-S_1 level.

Axial reconstruction (C, D, E, F), like computerized tomography, allows us to evaluate the features of the profile of the disc protrusion or any extrusion of the disc tissue.

In this case the axial reconstructions, cranio-caudally seriated at the level of the symptomatic disc (L_5-S_1), show a disc herniation which is extruded and migrated downwards, compressing and dislocating the nerve root at S_1 to the left.

It must be emphasized that magnetic resonance tomography is the only non-invasive method which permits exploration of the spine at the three spatial levels. In order to be able to obtain clear images the patient must be perfectly immobile, and the exploration field must be as small as possible.

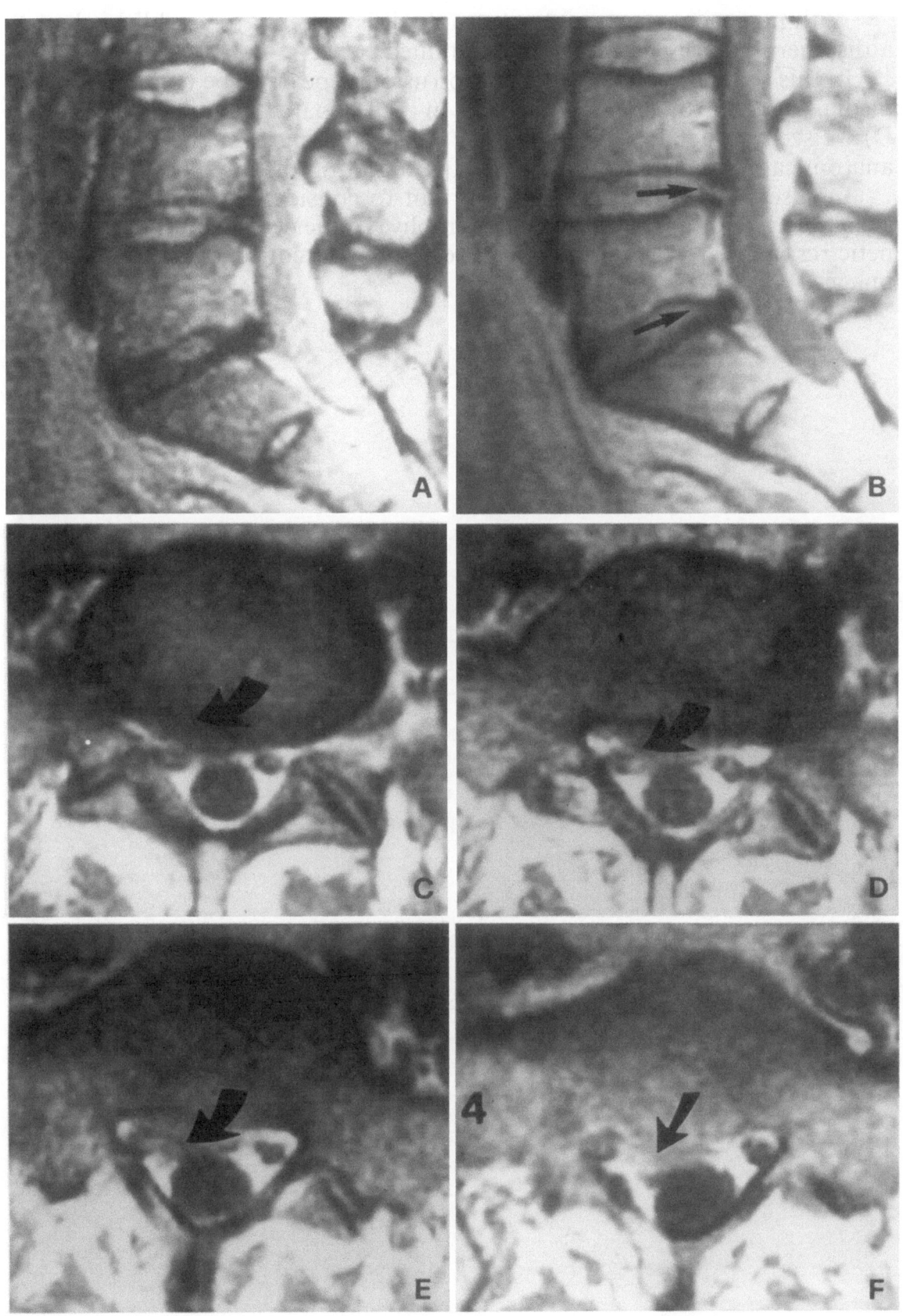

With magnetic resonance tomography it is not easy to establish whether a disc herniation is more or less contained.

In this series of images the disc protrusion appears to be contained in the medial sagittal projections (A, B), but in the left paramedian projections (C, D) we seem to be able to see the disc tissue running over the physiological anatomical margins and protruding by migrating distally.

In cases such as these, it is important to consider the following: I) the absolute need for intraoperative discography, II) the need to consider the magnetic resonance tomogram in its entirety, without concentrating on a single image.

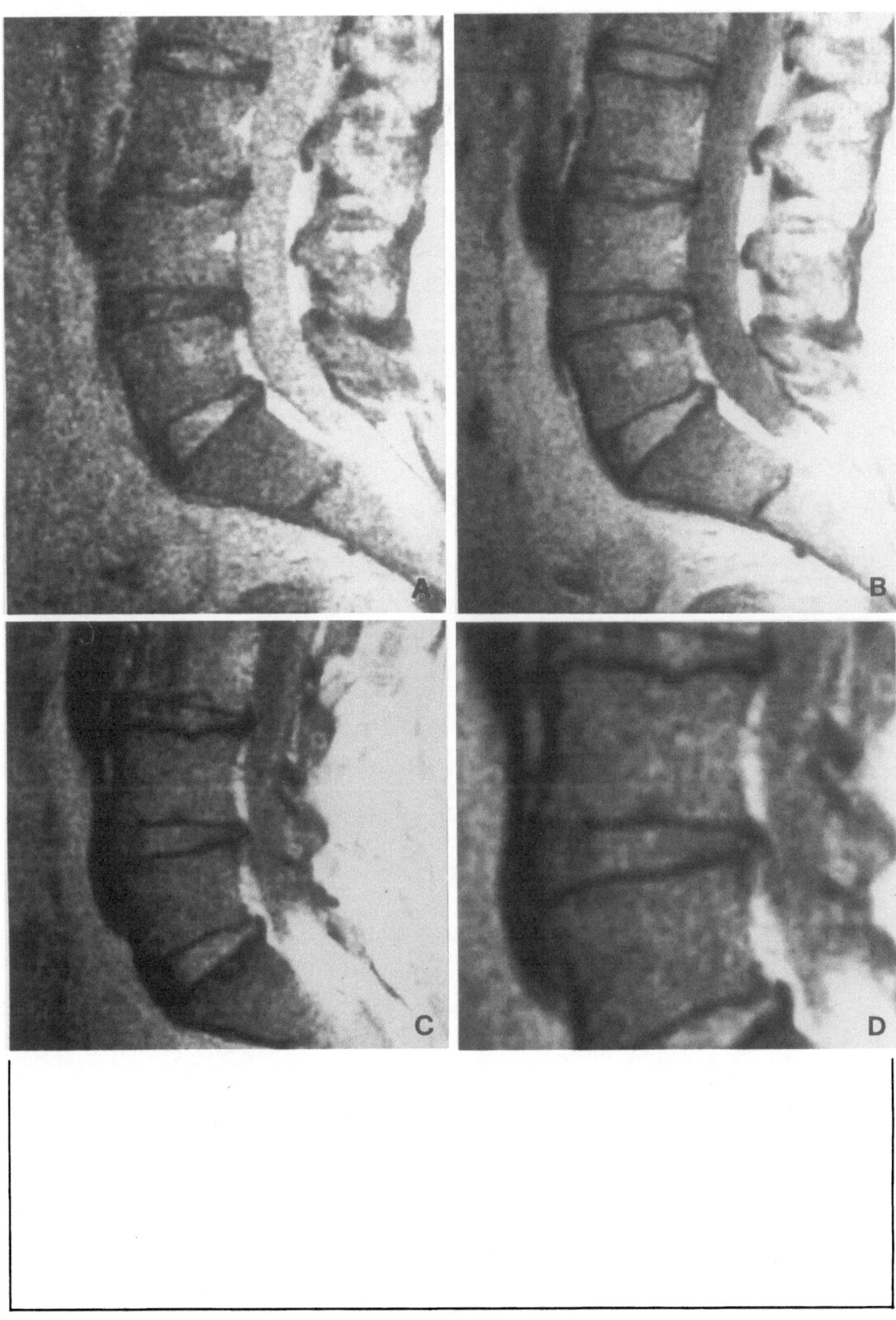

Only rarely are there pictures of disc herniation, which is clearly extruded, such as in this case (A, B, C) of disc hernation at L_5-S_1 in which the pulpy nucleus is totally projected in the vertebral canal, determining evident compression on the dural sac. Observe the discopathy located above L_4-L_5.

Percutaneous discectomy is clearly contraindicated in cases such as these.

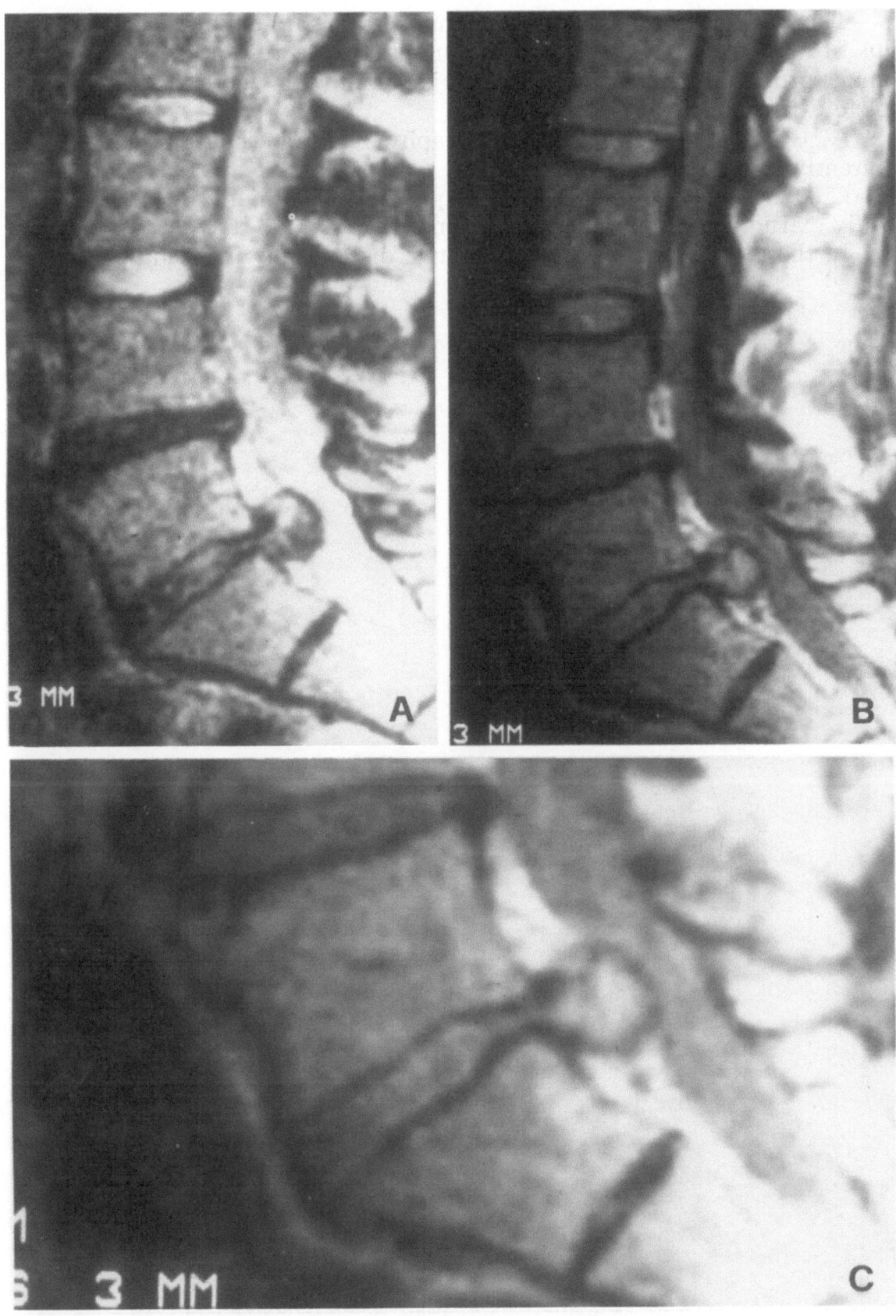

There is no evident criteria which may establish the integrity of the anulus fibrosus by magnetic resonance tomography, as resolution of the actual image processors and signal indicators is not allowed where there is no complete extrusion of the pulpy nucleus.

A, B) Magnetic resonance tomography of disc herniation at L_4-L_5, apparently contained.

C, D) Magnetic resonance tomography of disc herniation which is apparently extruded and migrated downwards.

In these cases, as well, intraoperative discography is essential.

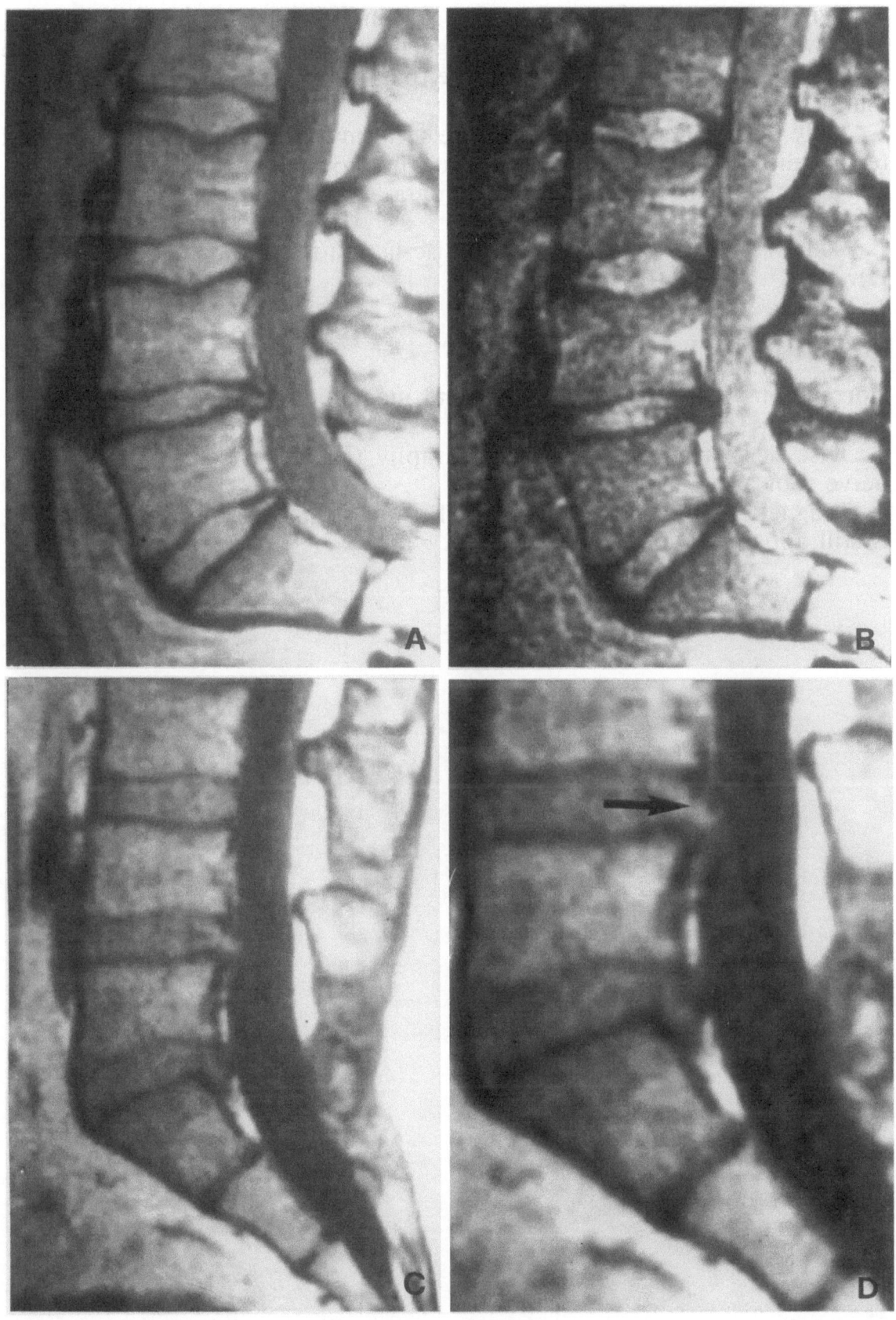

Symptomatic disc herniation at L_4-L_5 and asymptomatic discopathy at L_5-S_1 with disc protrusion (A, B). Magnetic resonance tomography tends to reveal several «disc herniations» more than those which are really symptomatic.

Only when there is a correspondence between clinical data and instrumental testing should we take an aggressive attitude to the treatment of the anomaly. Discrepancy between the clinical data and the image requires more in-depth diagnosis.

Axial reconstructions reveal the disc herniation between L_4 and L_5 (C, D).

Correlations between myelography and magnetic resonance tomography

Disc herniation at L_3-L_4. Myelography (E) lacks visualization of the nerve root at L_4 left.

Magnetic resonance tomography (F) shows that disc herniation at L_3-L_4 is still apparently contained.

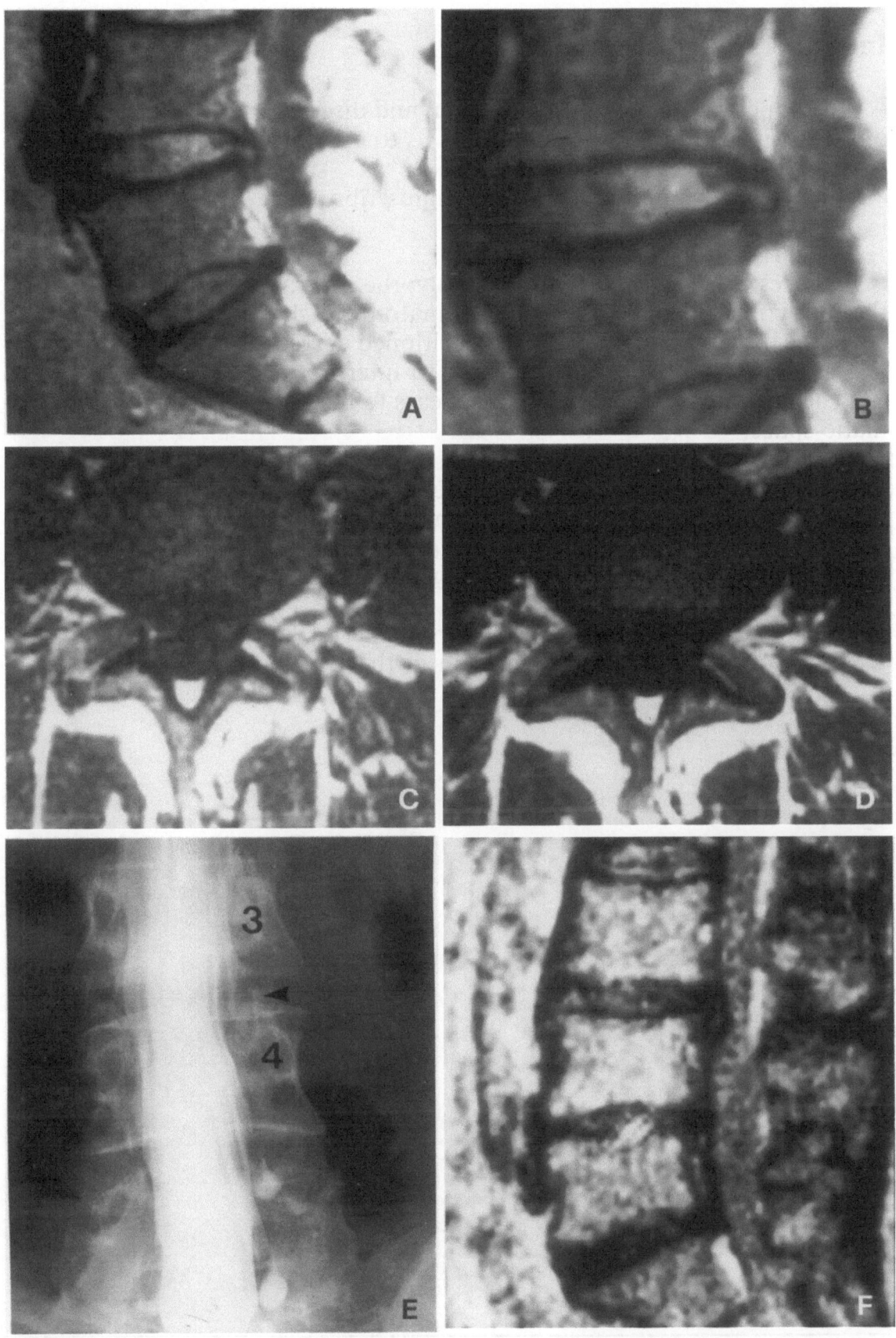

Intraoperative discography

Intraoperative discography is a final and discriminating test: it is carried out just before discectomy, and allows us to continue or end the procedure. It is the purpose of discography to:
— evaluate the integrity of the anulus fibrosus;
— reproduce the nerve root pain;
— carry out a discometry.

This test must be carried out correctly: the contrast medium must «paint» the pulpy nucleus and reproduce its anatomical shape (nucleography).

If the discography needle is not positioned correctly, there will be images of «anulography» which are difficult to interpret.

The healthy disc (A, B) always appears to be at the center of the intersomatic space.

The herniated disc is characterized by anular borders which in a latero-lateral projection run over the line of the posterior wall of the vertebral bodies, without showing overflow of contrast medium in the epidural space. In cases such as these the term «contained hernia» may be used, which may be treated according to the Onik method, as long as nerve root pain is evoked during the test.

C, D) «Contained» disc herniation at the L_5-S_1 level.
E, F) «Contained» disc herniation at the L_4-L_5 level.

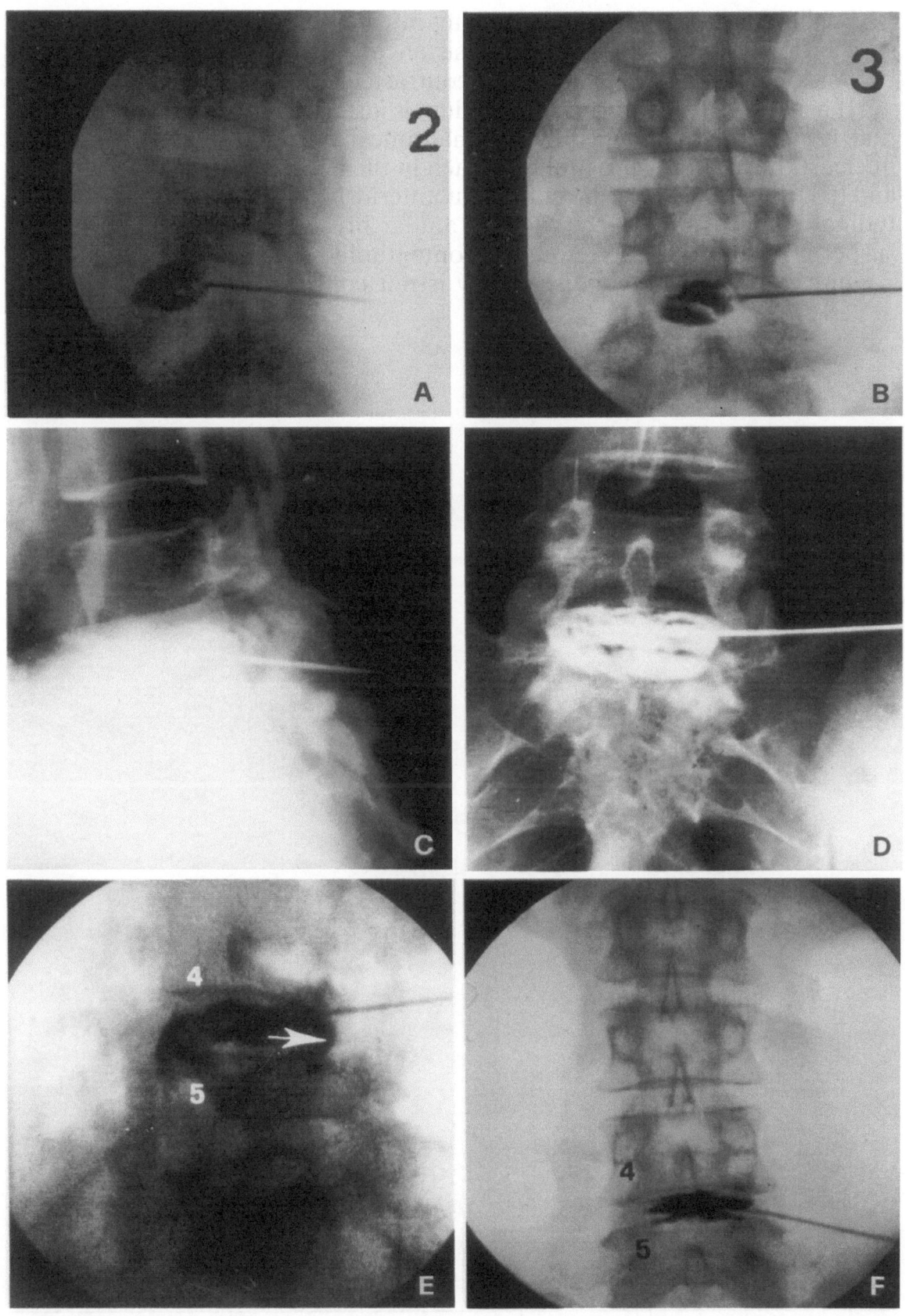

While the contrast medium is being injected into the pulpy nucleus the surgeon feels a certain amount of resistance which, if the anulus is whole, becomes incoercible after 2-4 cc of contrast medium have been injected.

If a larger quantity of contrast medium is instead easily injected, this means that it cannot be contained in the anatomical space destined to the pulpy nucleus: thus, there is probably a breach in the anular system. In figures (A) and (B) the contrast medium comes out anteriorly towards the anterior longitudinal ligament, revealing a ventral anular breach which could have been suspected with magnetic resonance tomography (C, D).

In cases such as these discectomy is not contraindicated.

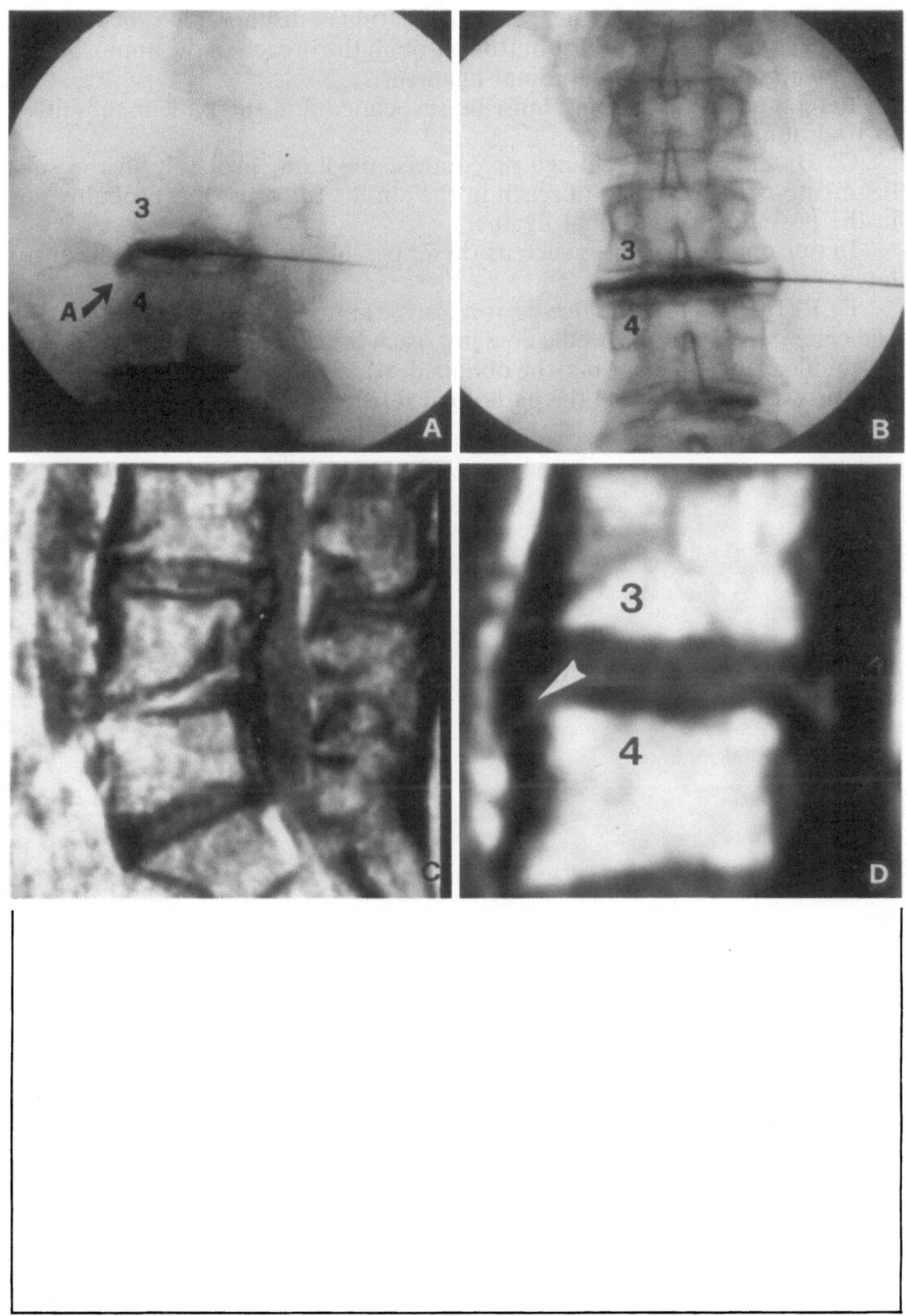

A, B) Clear image of typical extruded hernia at discography: the contrast medium comes out like a shirt button through the breach in the anulus fibrosus and the posterior longitudinal ligament.

Percutaneous discectomy must be suspended and the patient submitted to traditional surgery.

C, D) Linear escape image of contrast medium, probably in the subligamentous site: there is a breach in the anulus fibrosus, but probably not in the posterior longitudinal ligament.

In our opinion, in cases such as these, percutaneous discectomy is absolutely not contraindicated.

E, F) Insertion of the needle for discography requires extreme caution and care: if the tip of the needle does not reach the center of the pulpy nucleus, an «anulographic» image may be obtained, which is difficult to interpret and of little use in determining the pathological situation of «contained» or «extruded» hernia.

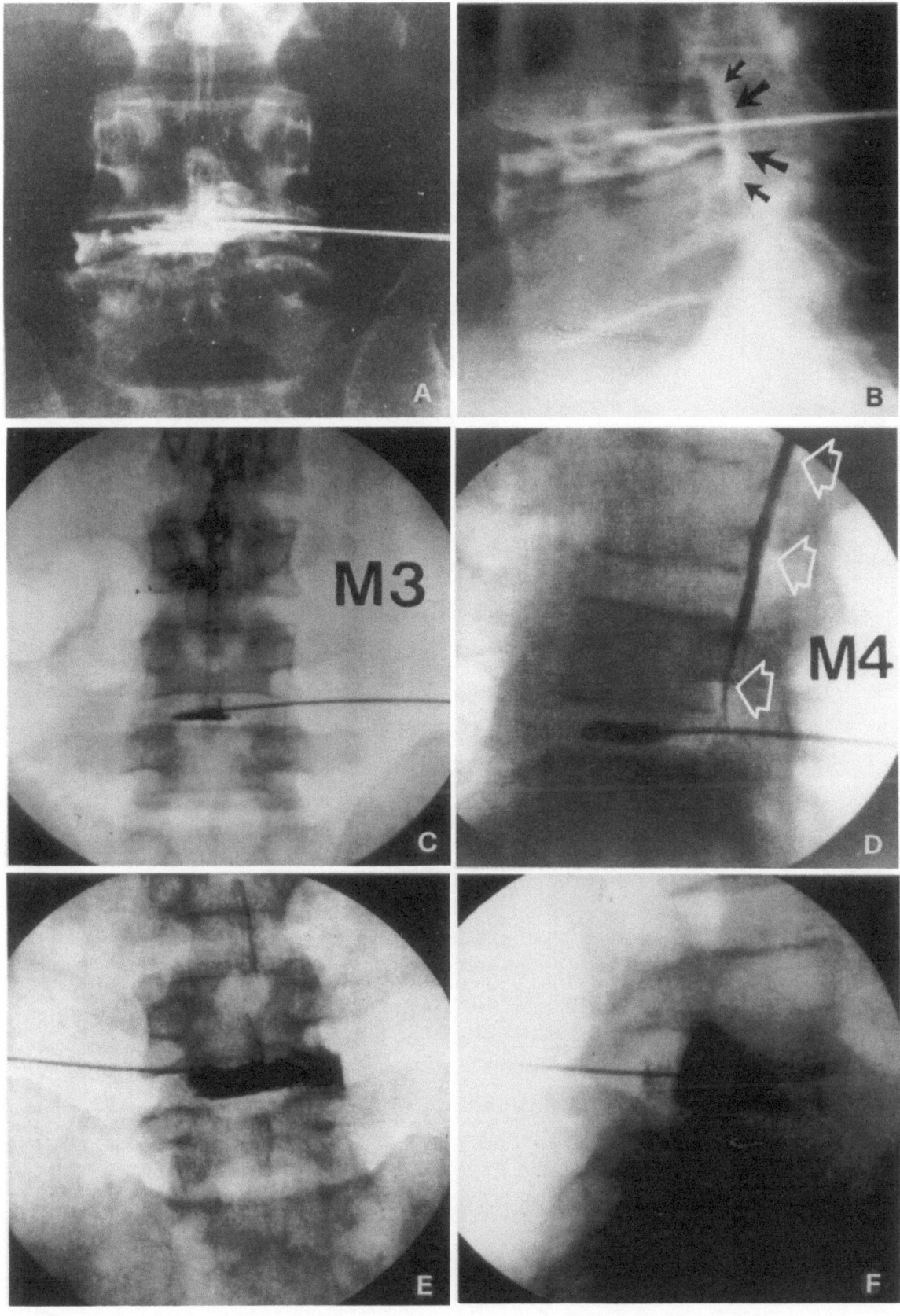

Surgical method
G. Orsini

— Instrumentation
— Stages of surgery

Instrumentation

The percutaneous discectomy system devised by Gary Onik is made up of a throw-away sterile kit, a console, and a recipient to collect the material which is aspired.

The first series of throw-away kits (C) was quite different from that being used at present (B); a guide (C) has been added, suitably curved to make the approach to the space at L_5-S_1 easier.

The throw-away kit groups together the various instruments, numbered according to the sequence in which they are used; furthermore, it comes with a dermatographic pencil, an osteotome, a decimeter, and a syringe which, inserted into the appropriate three-way faucet, may de-obstruct the aspiration tube, if necessary.

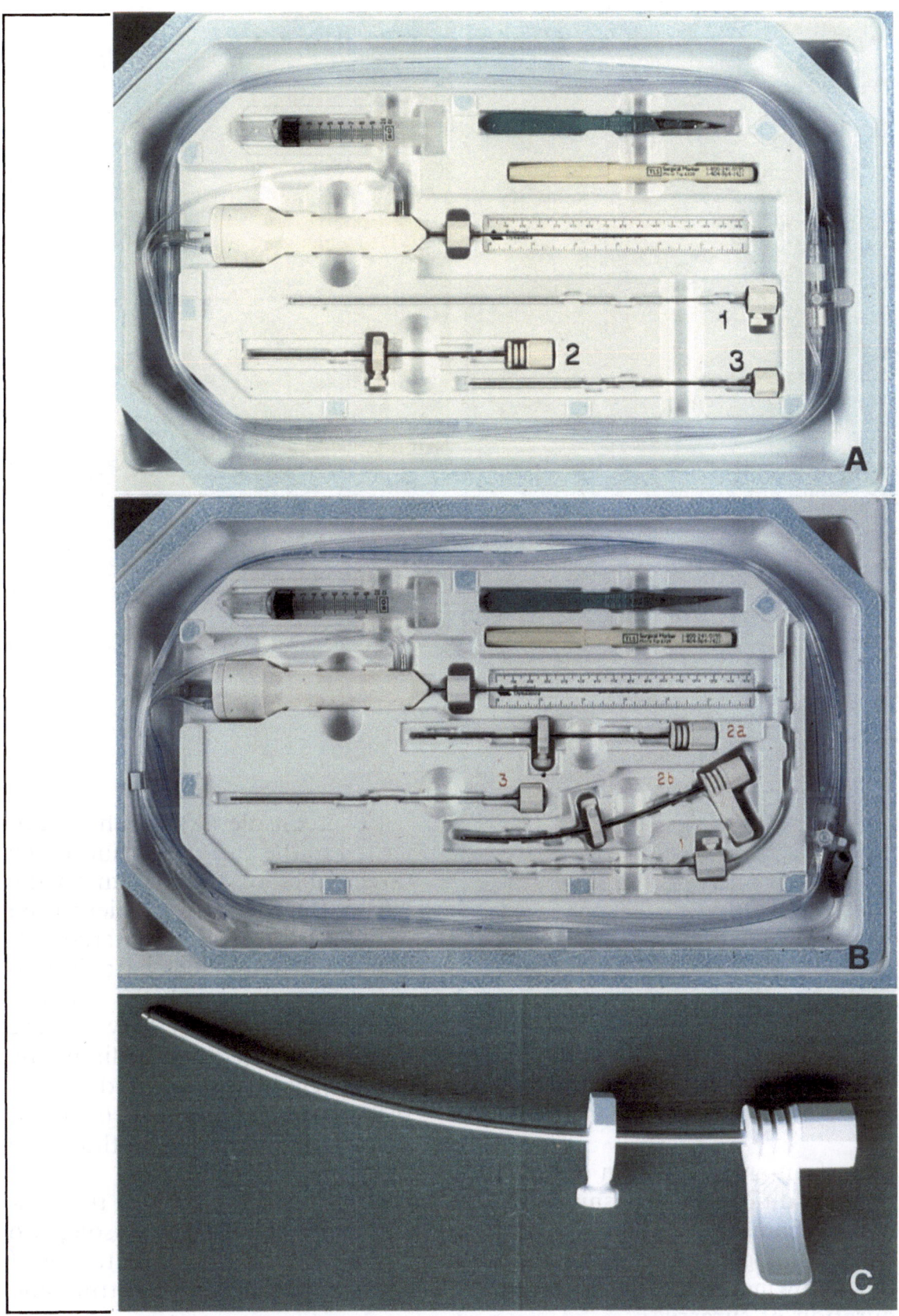

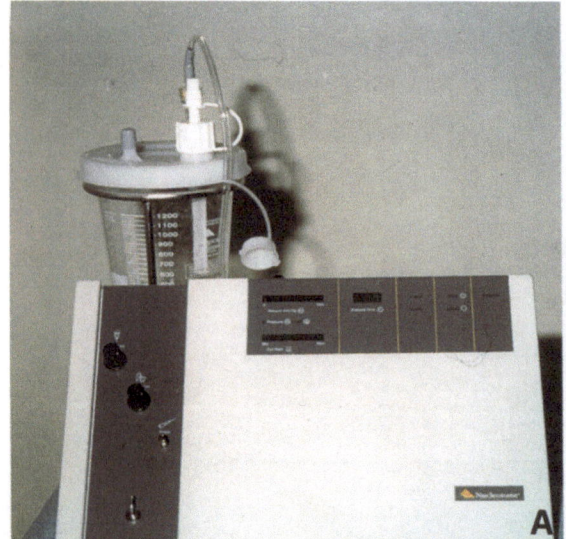

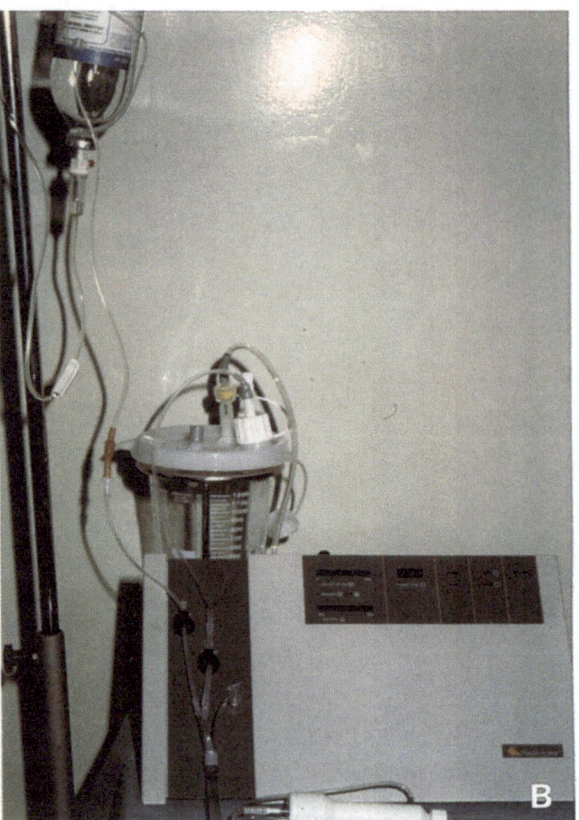

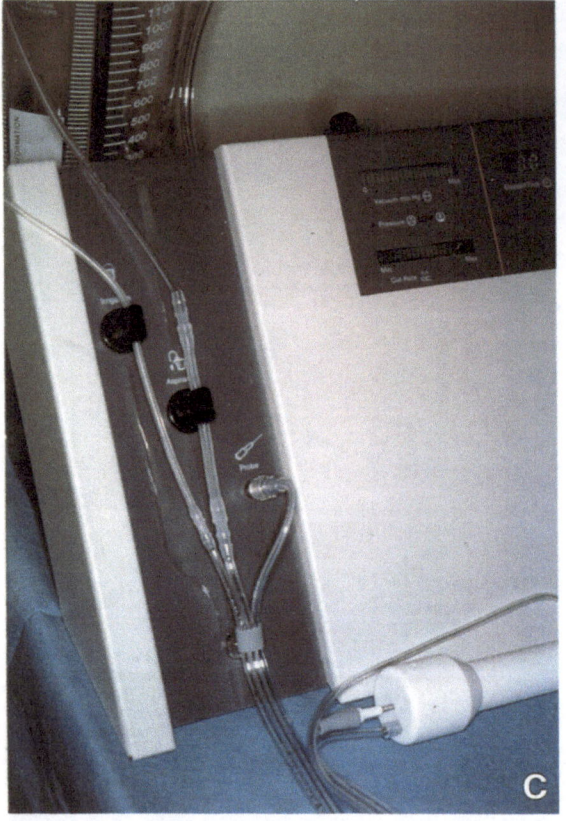

The console (A) which is connected to the current, connects the three tubes of the system to the lavage fluid, to the recipient used to collect the aspired material (B), and to the pump. The latter is activated by stepping on the pedal.

The connections between the various tubes (C) are facilitated by the fastening system, and by the fact that they are of different lengths and diameters; thus, the risk of an error in union is practically impossible.

In addition to the flashing lights providing information on how the various mechanisms are functioning, there are three displays on the console, two of the analogic type and one of the digital type, allowing for monitoring of the following: negative pressure of the recipient, frequency of cutting and duration of surgery.

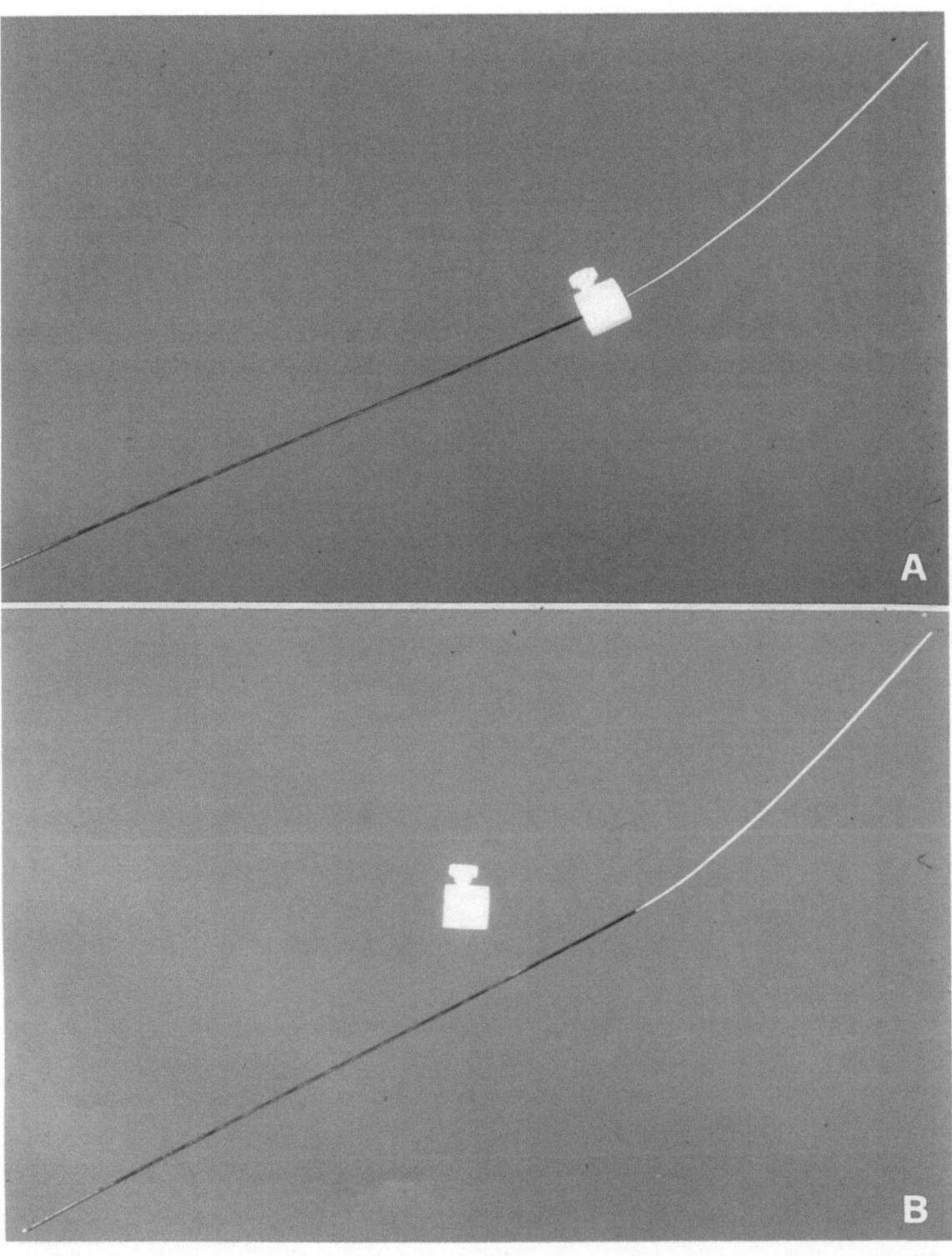

The instrument (A) marked on the kit box with a n. 1 is the wireguide (1 mm in diameter) which is inserted in the intervertebral disc to be operated. Once it has been positioned in the correct site, it is released by the small handle (B) so that the successive instruments may be introduced, which will thus be correctly piloted.

Instrument 2a is constituted by two coaxial cannulae (A): of these, the more external one (sheath) has a diameter of 2.6 mm and is provided with a small handle with a bayonetlike clutch and a disc which may slide freely, and which will act as a cutaneous arrest.

The smaller cannula (dilator) is an empty cylinder 2 mm in diameter which, after the sheath has been fastened by the bayonetlike clutch, helps to dilate the various tissues to be crossed (B). Its extremity, slightly conical and cutting, protrudes from the sheath by 2 mm (C) so as to produce a circular trace on the surface of the anulus fibrosus, thus keeping the next instrument from «slipping».

In fact, let us recall that for the entire duration of the operation the sheath is always only leaned up against the anulus and not fastened to it.

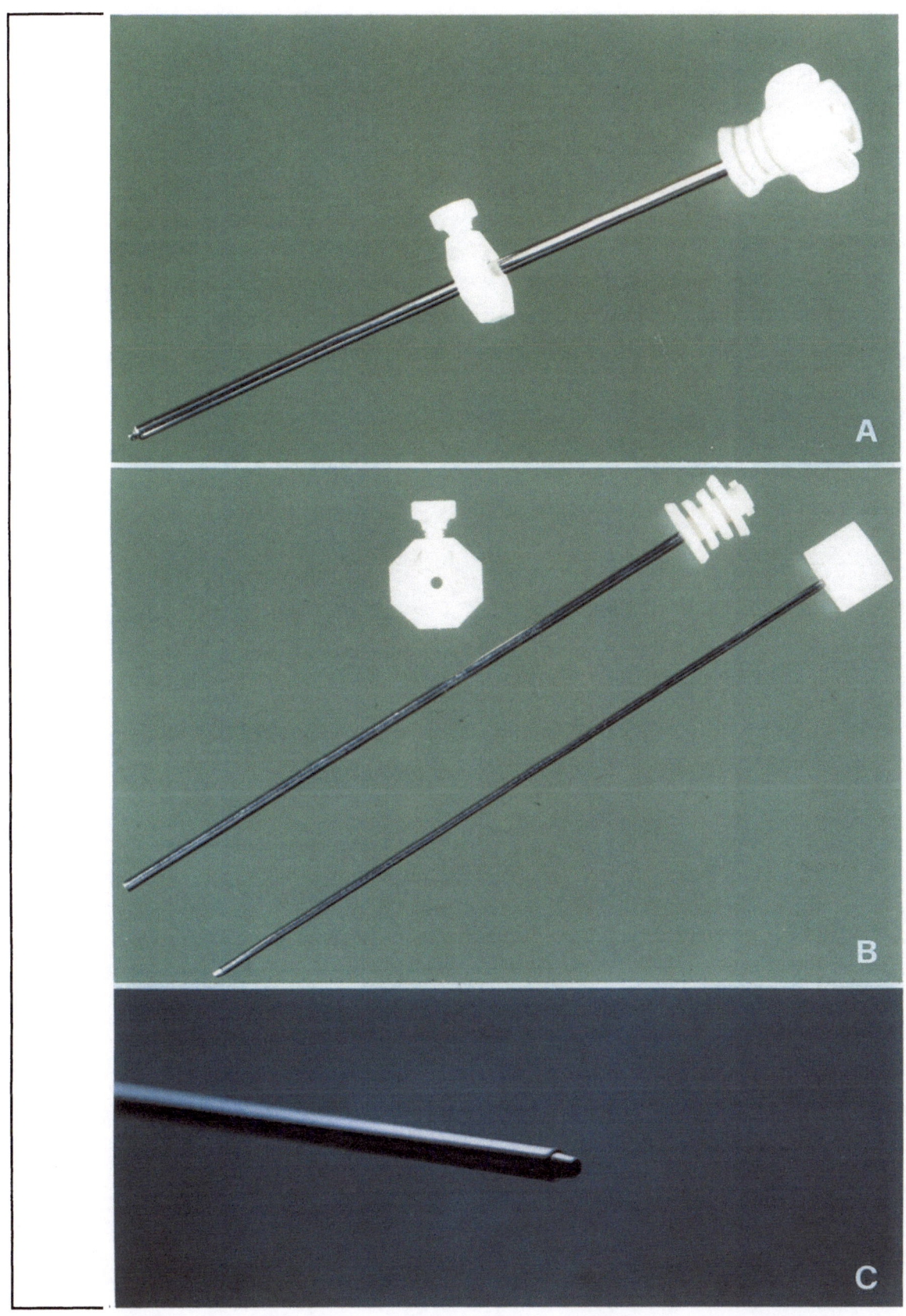

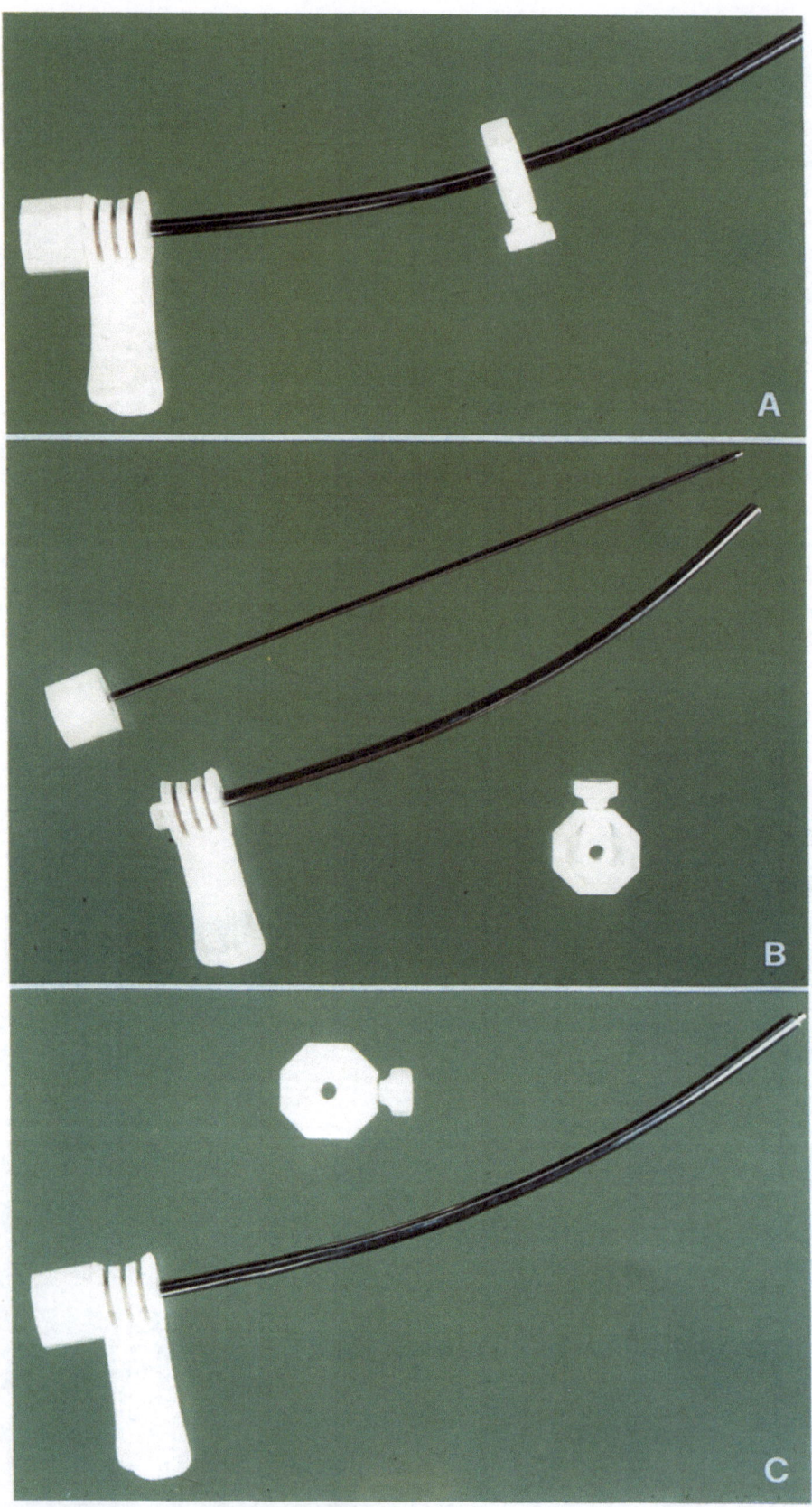

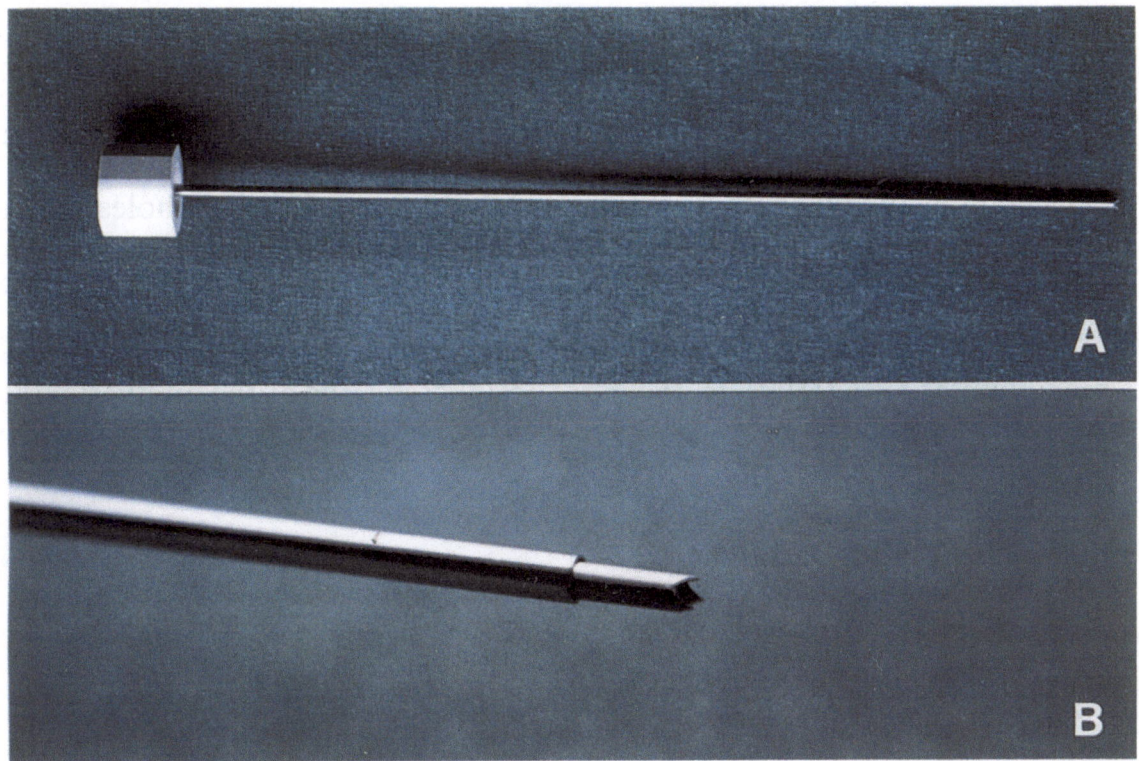

The n. 3 instrument is the anulus-breaker (A): it consists in a cannula 2 mm in diameter, provided with a small handle, having a cutting, saw-toothed edge.

After the dilator has been extracted, the anulus-breaker is inserted in its place in the sheath. As the latter protrudes 8 mm (B) a hole of equal length and 2 mm in diameter, allowing for free access to the pulpy nucleus, may be made in the anulus fibrosus.

◄

The curved sheath is marked 2b (A), and it is used to obtain easier access to the L_5-S_1 space when the iliac crest produces a skeletal obstacle before the intervertebral disc.

This anatomical situation occurs in 82% of the population for the L_5-S_1 space, but we must not overlook the fact that in 8% of the cases the L_4-L_5 space is also difficult to reach with straight instruments.

Moreover, it must be emphasized that, apart from the sheaths, which are rigid, all of the other instruments may be adapted to the curvature ray of the instrument marked 2b (B, C).

The probe, or actual nucleotome, is made up of a cannula 2 mm in diameter, connected to a handle which encloses the entire pneumatic mechanism for the cutter and the circulation paths for the lavage fluid (A). ▶

A ferrule slides on the cannula, which is connected by its bayonetlike clutch to the handle of the sheath.

The end of the nucleotome is rounded and has small lateral holes 2 mm x 2 mm, within which one may see the blade of the cutter move up and down (B, C), working with a guillotine like movement: through this hole the disc material is aspired and fragmented.

The end of the cannula of the nucleotome sticks out of the sheath for a maximum of 3 cm (D): thus, the more peripheral areas of the intervertebral disc may be reached.

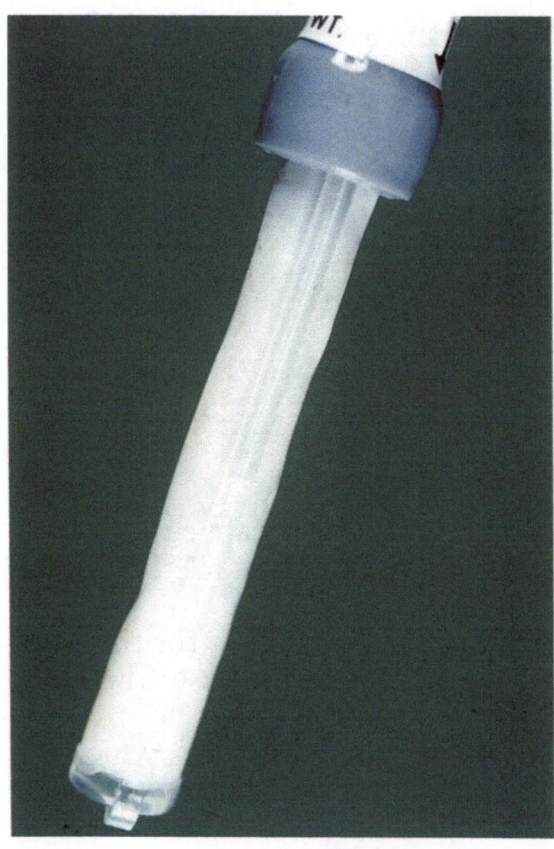

Inside the recipient which collects the drainage-lavage fluid, and which works as a vacuum, there is a filtrating test-tube, inside which the chips of disc material are kept, proof that discectomy has occurred.

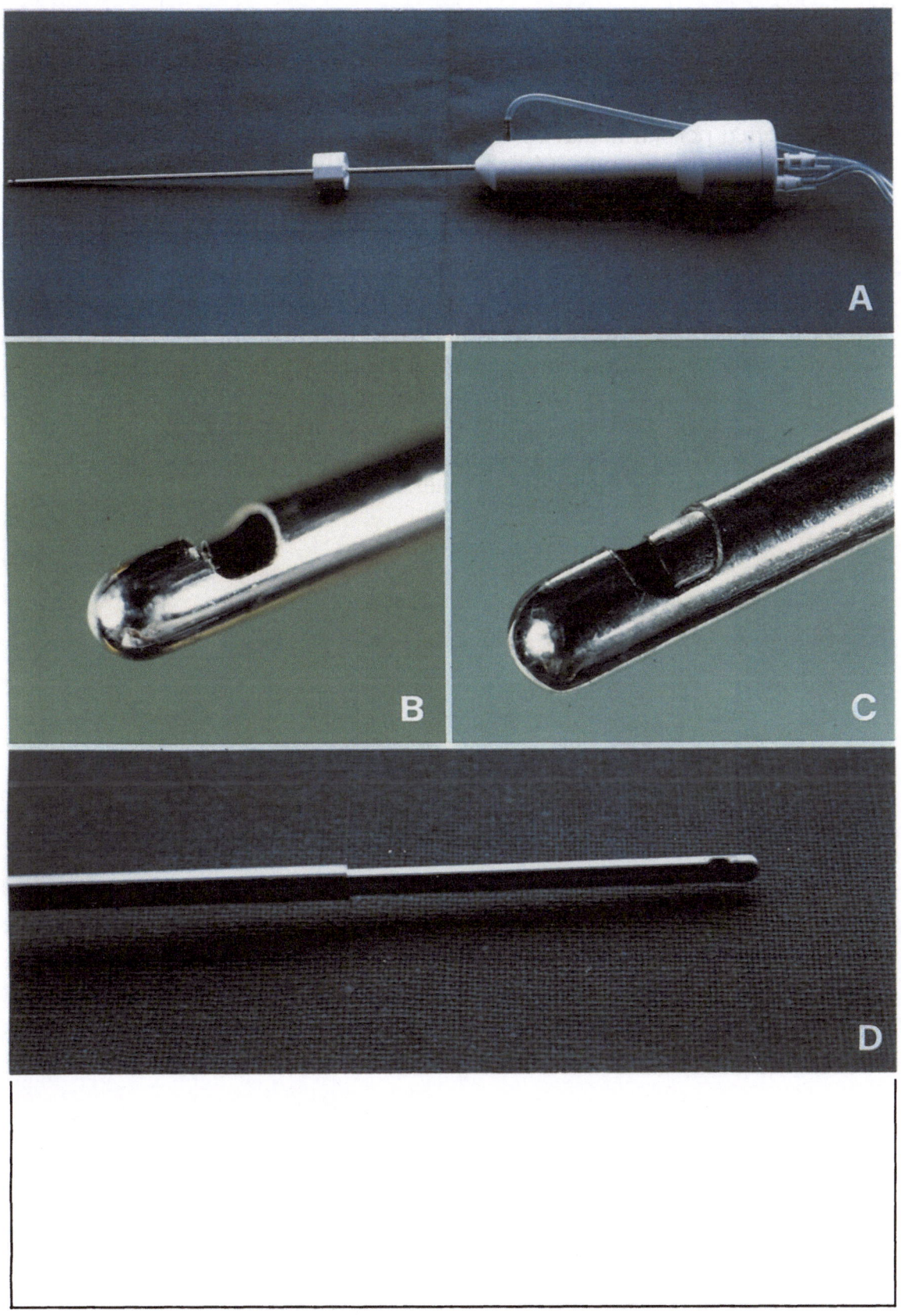

Stages of surgery

Prior to surgery a panoramic computerized tomography must *always* be obtained of the abdomen with the patient in a prone position and with the gantry directed perpendicular to the support plane at the level of the disc to be submitted to discectomy (A). This test firstly allows us to exclude the presence of retropsoic colic loops, which would be interposed in the passage of the instrumentation. This occurrence is described in 4% of the population, and it is best to recall that when a colic loop is accidentally penetrated secondary anaerobic discitis may occur.

Panoramic computerized tomography also reveals the anatomical disc center, which is located at the union between the posterior third and the anterior two thirds of the somatic plate (B), and establishes the inclination angle of the path to be made by the instruments (C).

Taking advantage of the centimetric scale located above and to the right on the tomogram, the distance from the insertion site to the line of the spinosae may be approximately measured on the skin.

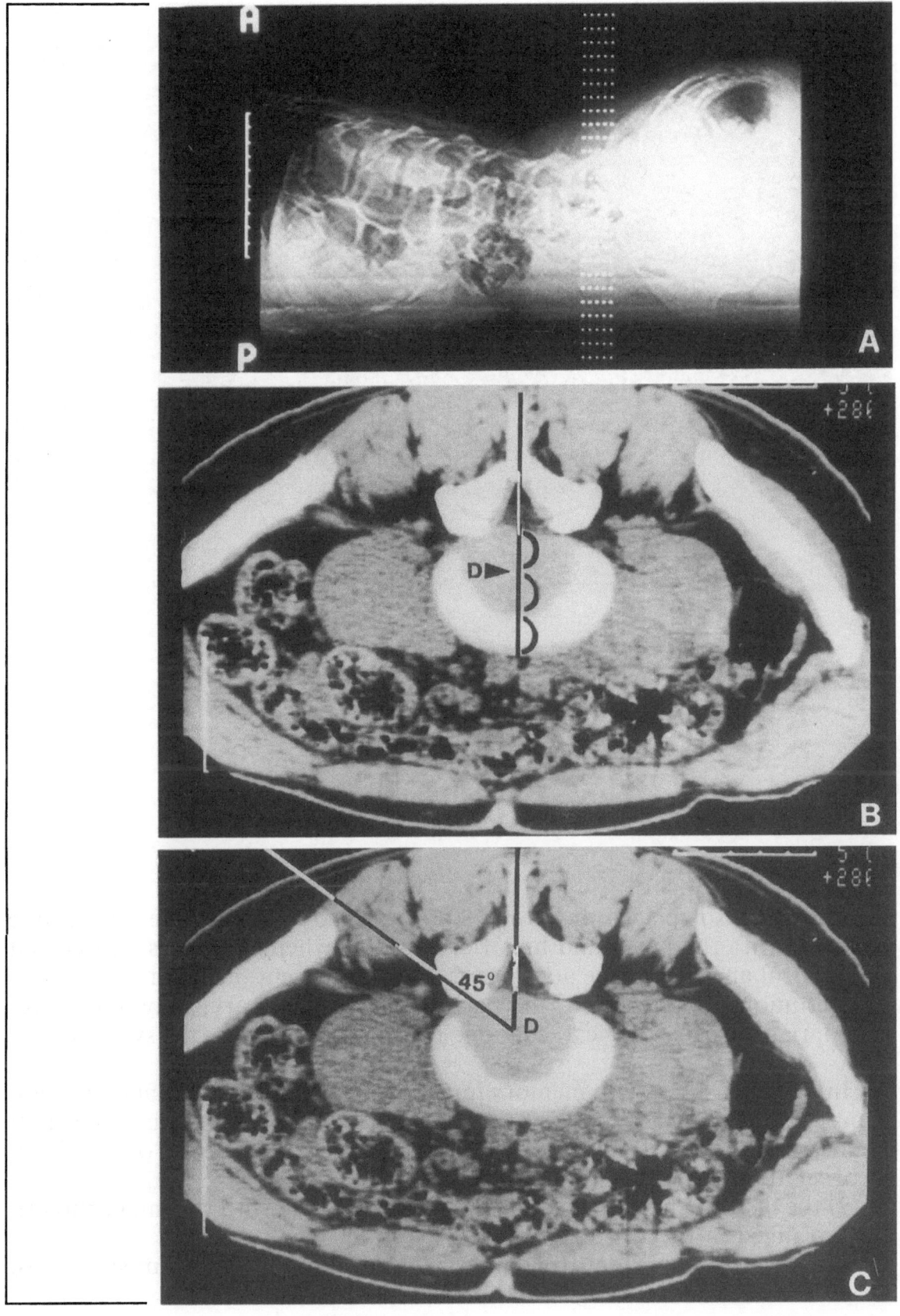

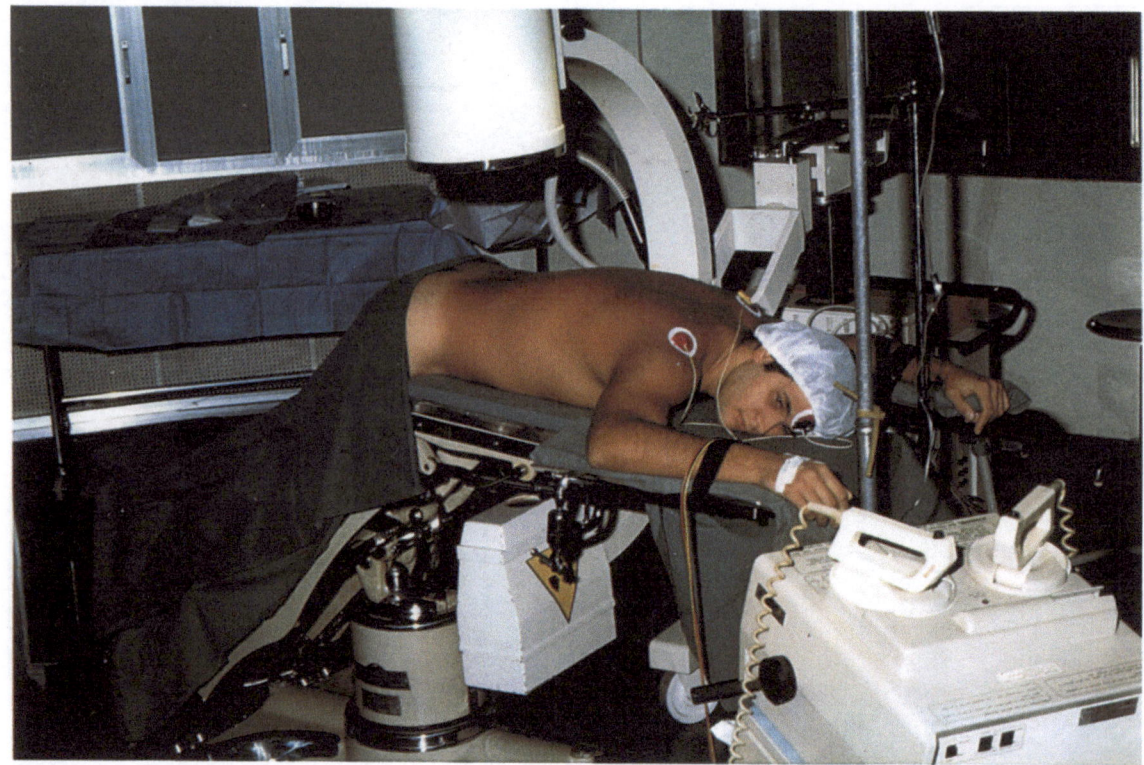

The patient is placed on a radiotransparent operating table, in a prone position, with the knees and hips flexed. Even when surgery is carried out under local anesthesia, the anesthesist *must* be present, as he or she will see to continuous monitoring of the patient, and if necessary, may administer appropriate pharmacological sedation. The approach is from the symptomatic side.

Image intensifier, with memory image videos, is placed so that on request it may provide images in A-P and L-L projections, keeping in mind that:

1) the images must show the disc being operated at the center of the video, in order to avoid errors in parallaxis;

2) the instrumentation must be inserted beginning with the image intensifier arranged in the L-L projection.

Finally, it is important to emphasize that all operating room staff must be protected from ionizing radiation by special aprons.

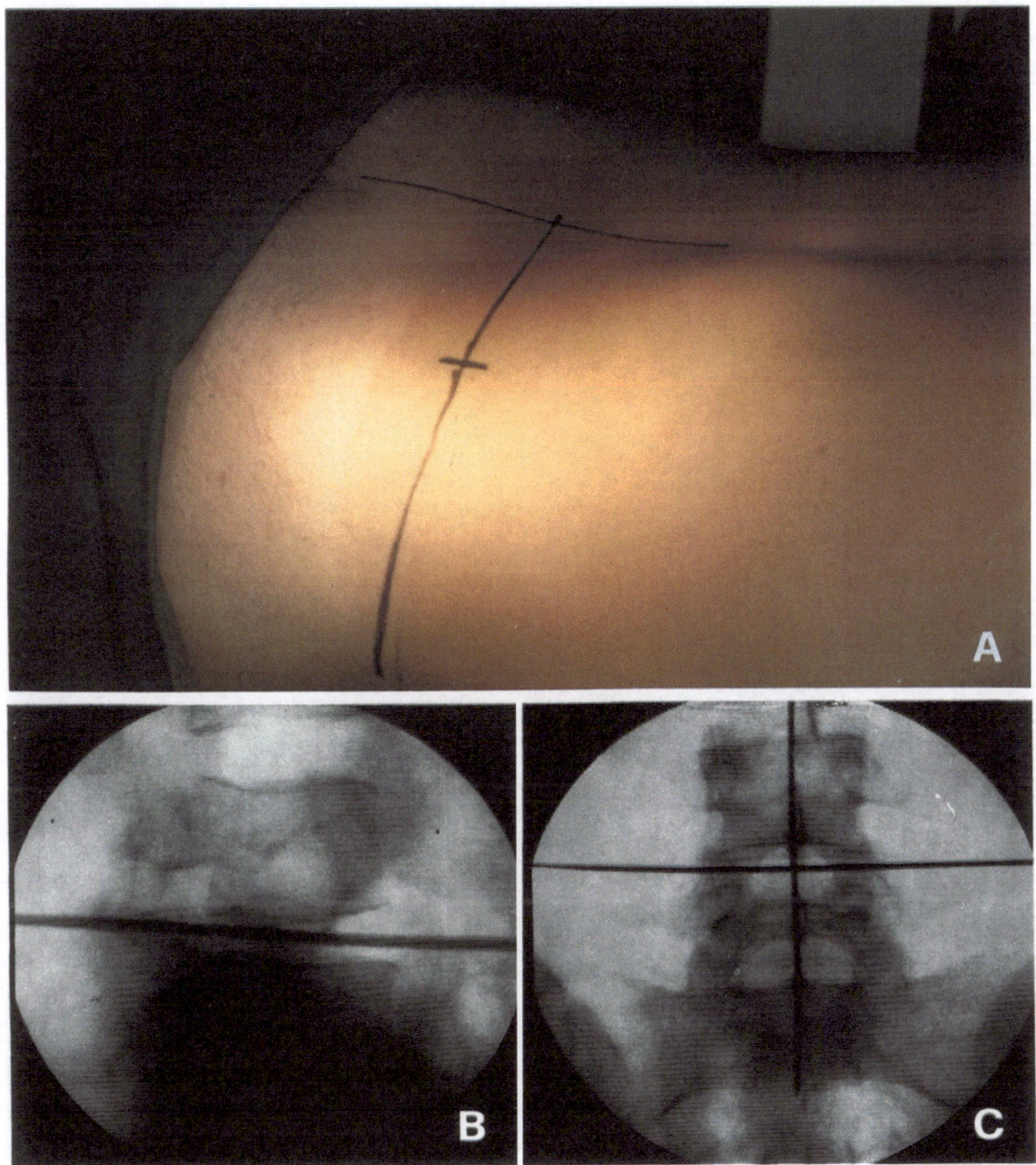

Using a dermatographic pencil and under radioscopic monitoring, the coordinates of the line of the spinous processes and of the disc space (A) are traced, and on the latter the entry site of the instrumention, which was measured previously on the panoramic computerized tomogram, is marked.

When we know the two orthogonal coordinates (B, C) as well as the insertion angle (page 85, C) it is easier to reach the intervertebral disc. These coordinates must be marked on the skin with a metallic reference point which may even be a simple Kirschner wire.

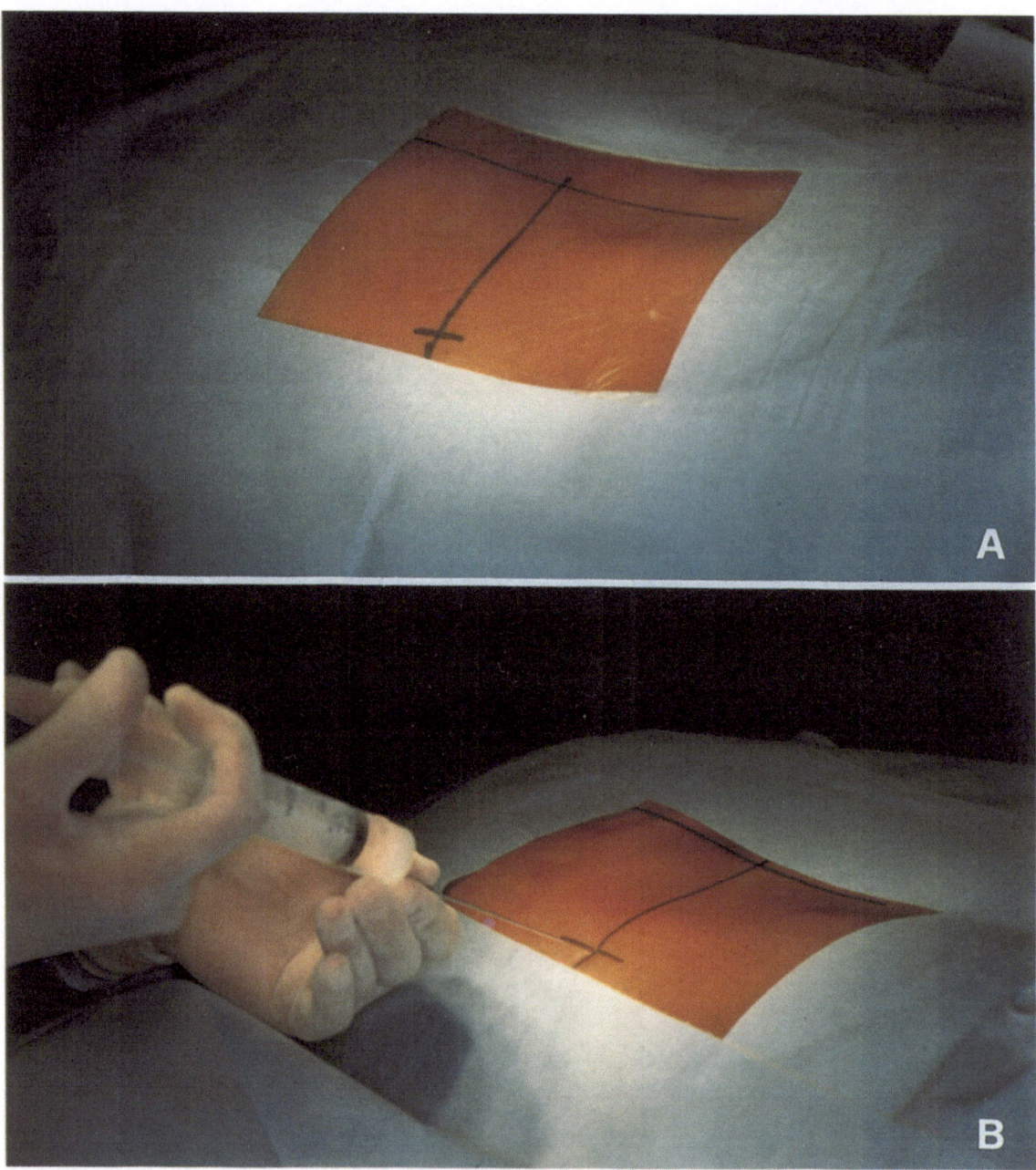

We now proceed to prepare the surgical field (A), following all of the rules of the most rigorous asepsis; local anesthesia is carried out (B) infiltrating the skin, subdermis and muscles as far as the joint facets, using a spinal injection needle.

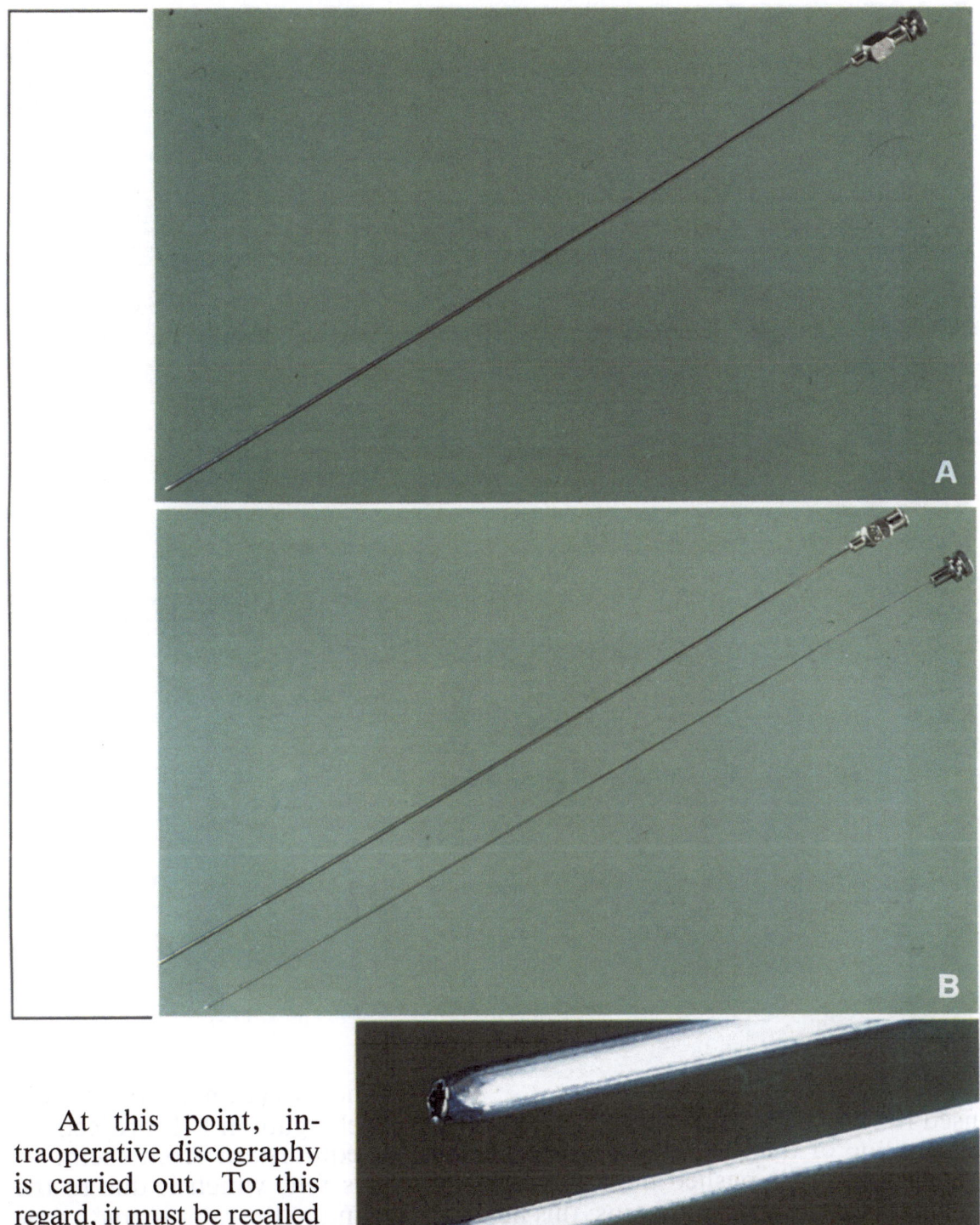

At this point, intraoperative discography is carried out. To this regard, it must be recalled that the discography needle (A) (19 g x 8 1/2'' mod.) has a spindle (B) the tip of which (C) must be like a javelin and not a mouthpiece. This is important because if the tip should be like a mouthpiece it could deviate the needle from its path as it crosses the various anatomical formations.

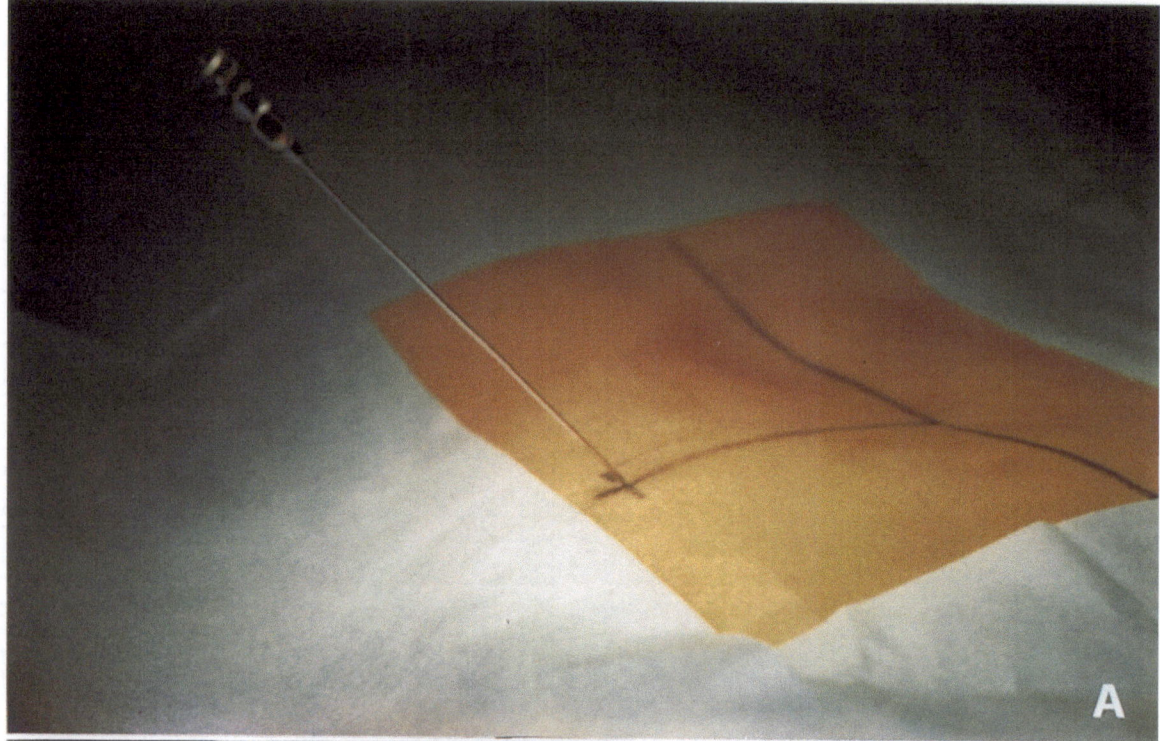

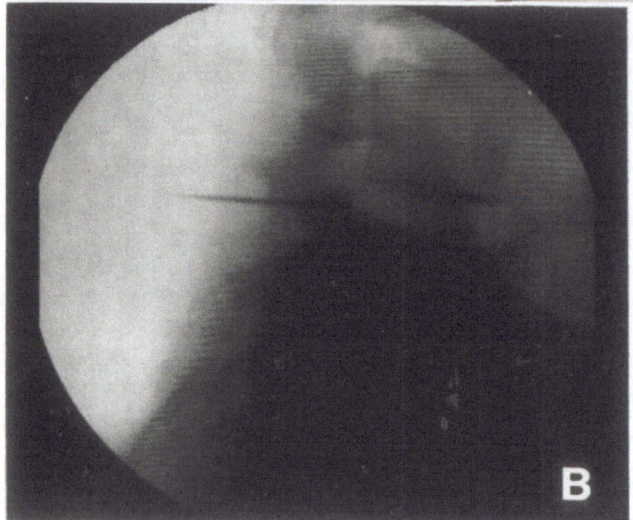

The direction of the needle used for discography (A) must be perfectly parallel, again in L-L projection, to the line of the somatic vertebral plates, and equidistant from them.

The needle is pushed until elastic resistance is felt, which is due to the contact with the anulus fibrosus; this must correspond to the radioscopic image in L-L projection (B) of the tip of the needle in the site of the posterior margin of the vertebral bodies.

The spindle is extracted from the needle, and a syringe is used for aspiration: in this manner, there is no injury to the radicular veins, an event which would produce retropsoic haematoma, which may even be of considerable size, and visualized by TRM.

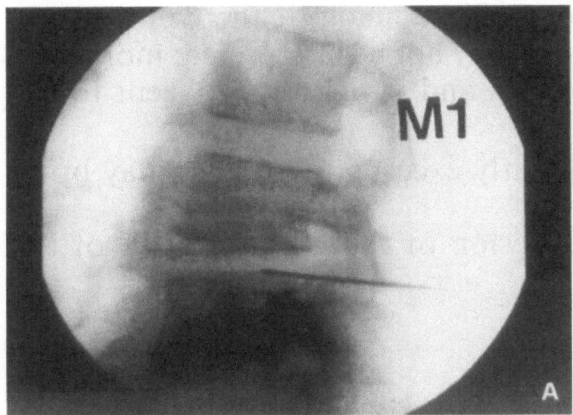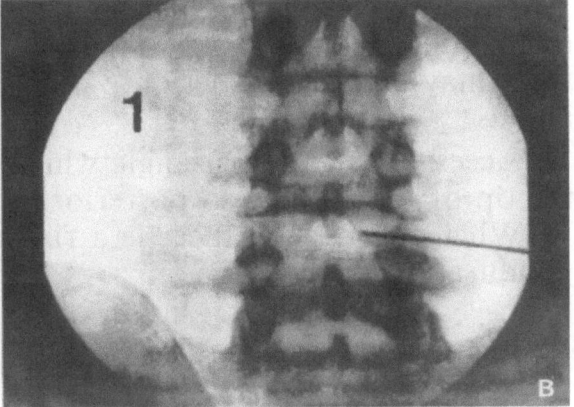

After penetrating into the intervertebral disc, in order to check that the needle is in the correct position, the radioscopic image must be referred to in its two standard orthogonal projections, which must show the following:

1) in L-L the needle contained in the posterior third of the disc area (A);

2) in A-P the tip of the needle does not surpass a line tangent to the medial border of the vertebral pedicle, a line which is considered to constitute the external limit of the dural sac encumbrance (B).

If these rules are not followed, errors will be made; if the contrast medium infiltrates the anulus fibrosus, the test may not be interpreted; moreover, there may be a risk of lesion of the organs and structures adjacent to the anulus.

Access with an upper angle which greatly exceeds 45 degrees may bring the tip of the needle too posterior.

When this occurs, there is a risk of lesion of the dural sac and of the peridural vein plexuses.

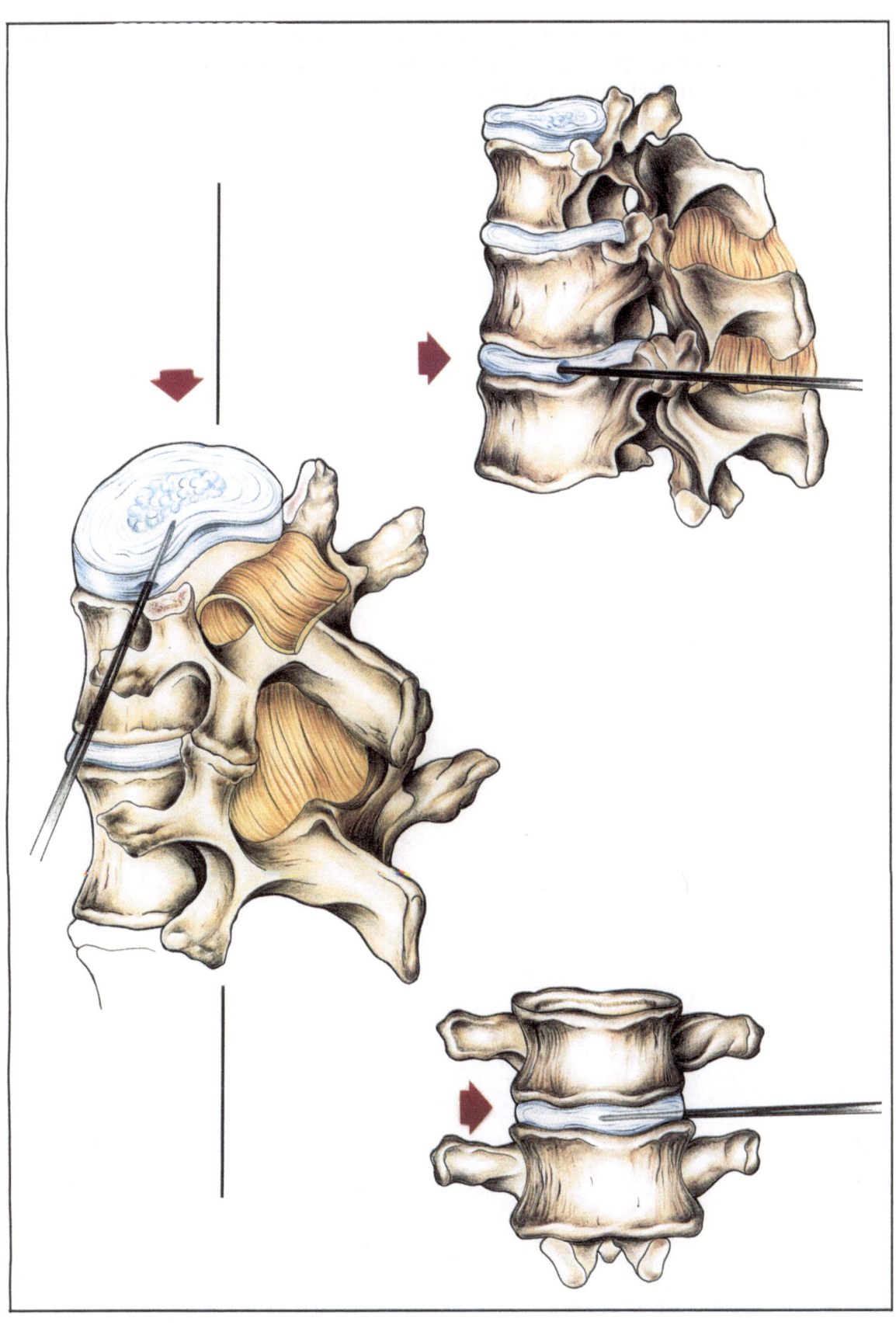

On the contrary, access with a penetration angle measuring less than 45 degrees may bring the tip of the needle too anterior, and thus produce a potential risk of lesion of the large vessels.

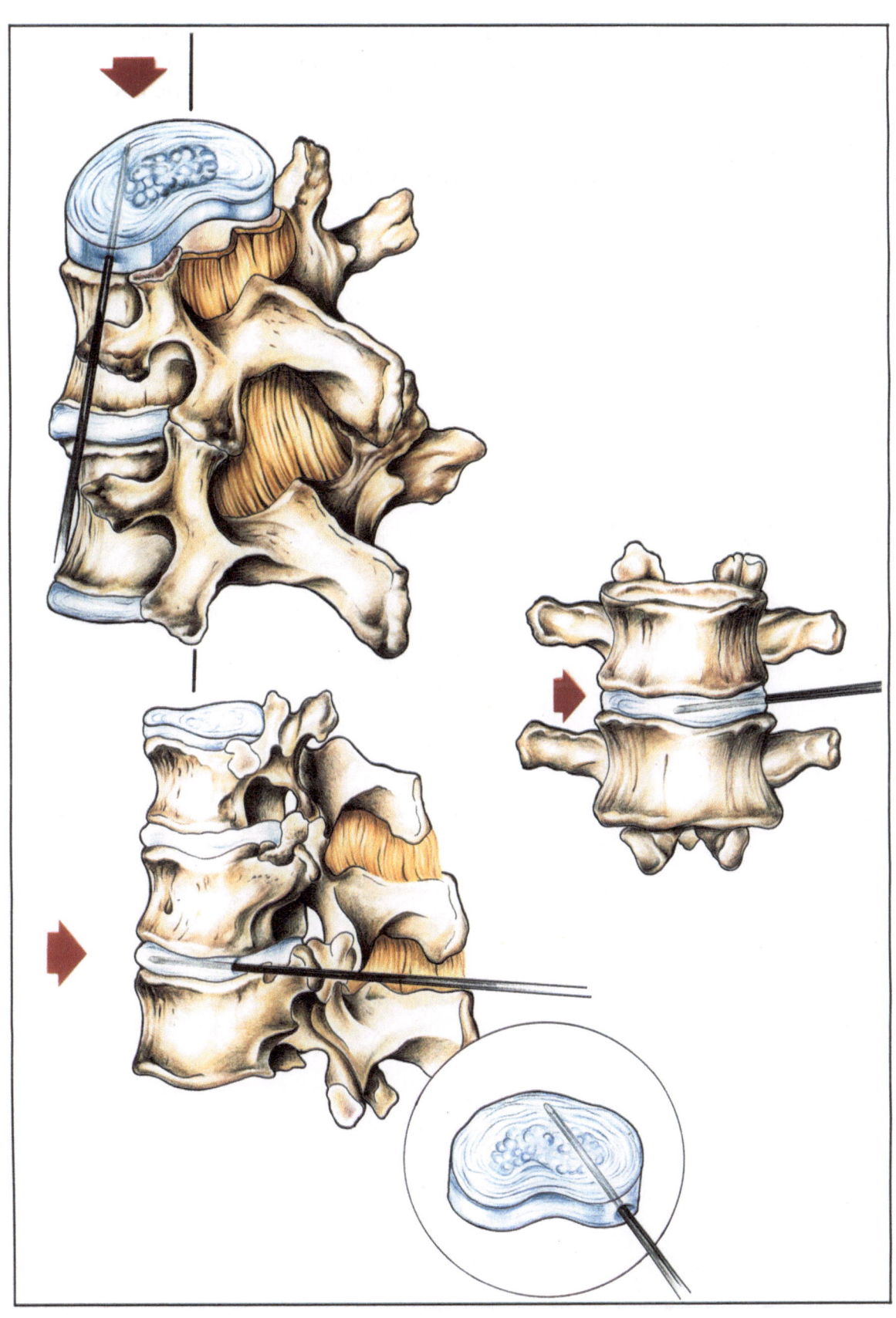

In cases where the approach is to the disc spaces in which the iliac alae constitute an obstacle difficult to overcome, it is best to resort to a curved sheath (marked n. 2b in the kit), which was recently added to the instrumentation.

Let us recall that skeletal obstacles, in addition to the iliac alae, may be constituted by a hyperplasia of the transverse processes or of the interapophysary processes.

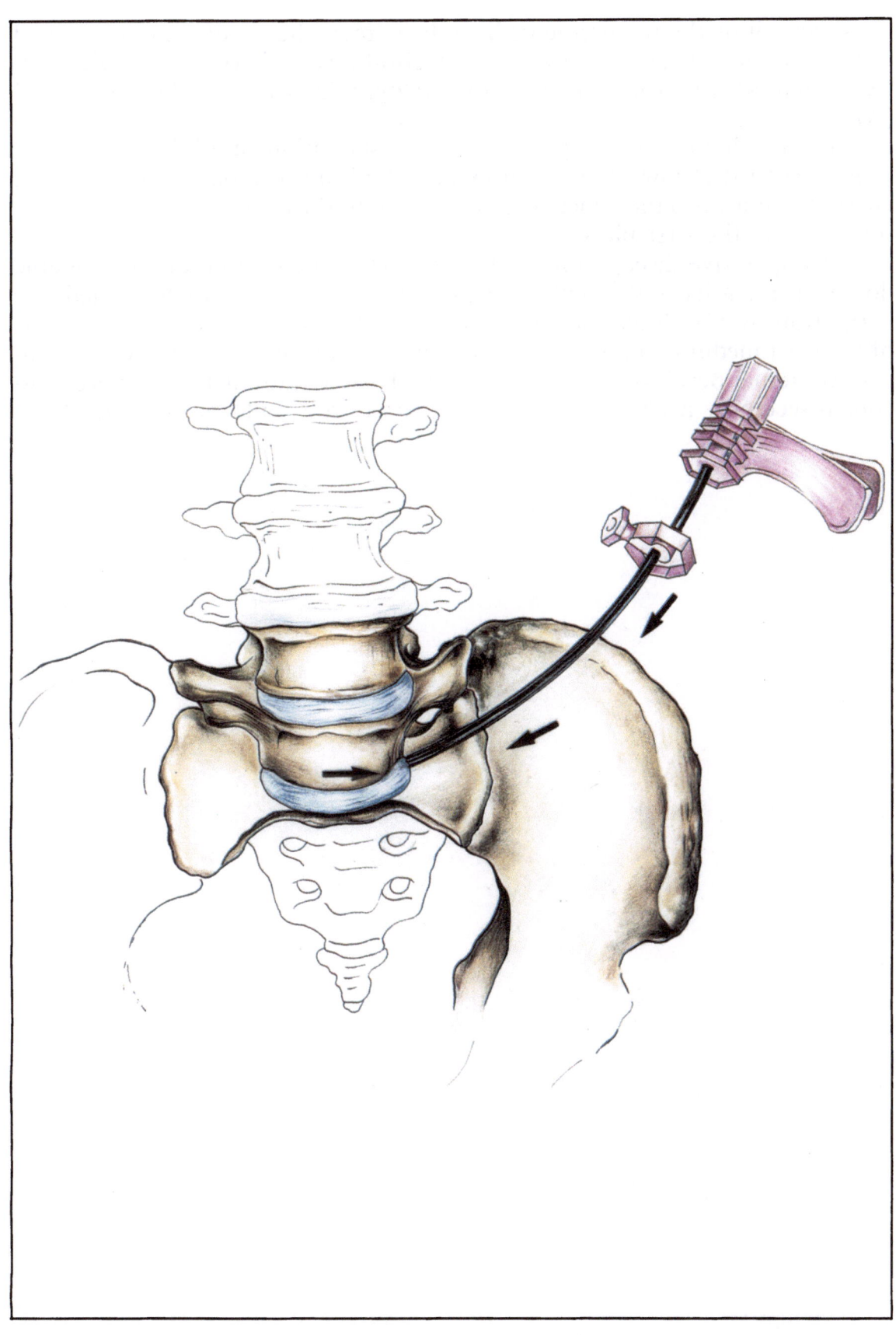

When all of the requirements have been met, the needle may be moved to the anatomical center of the intervertebral disc and contrast medium injected, that which is routinely used for myelography (hydrosoluble, non-ionic) (A).

The introduction of contrast medium must continue until there is evident resistence to the flow of the radiopaque fluid and the patient under local anesthesia must feel the typical pain irradiated to the lower leg which required treatment in the first place.

Intraoperative discography will help to evaluate beyond any reasonable doubt the integrity of the anulus fibrosus and thus the state of contained disc herniation (B, C). When the test for pain is negative, or when there is a loss of contrast medium in the vertebral canal, which in some cases provides images of actual peridurography (D, E), the basic requirements for percutaneous discectomy are not met, and the procedure should be suspended.

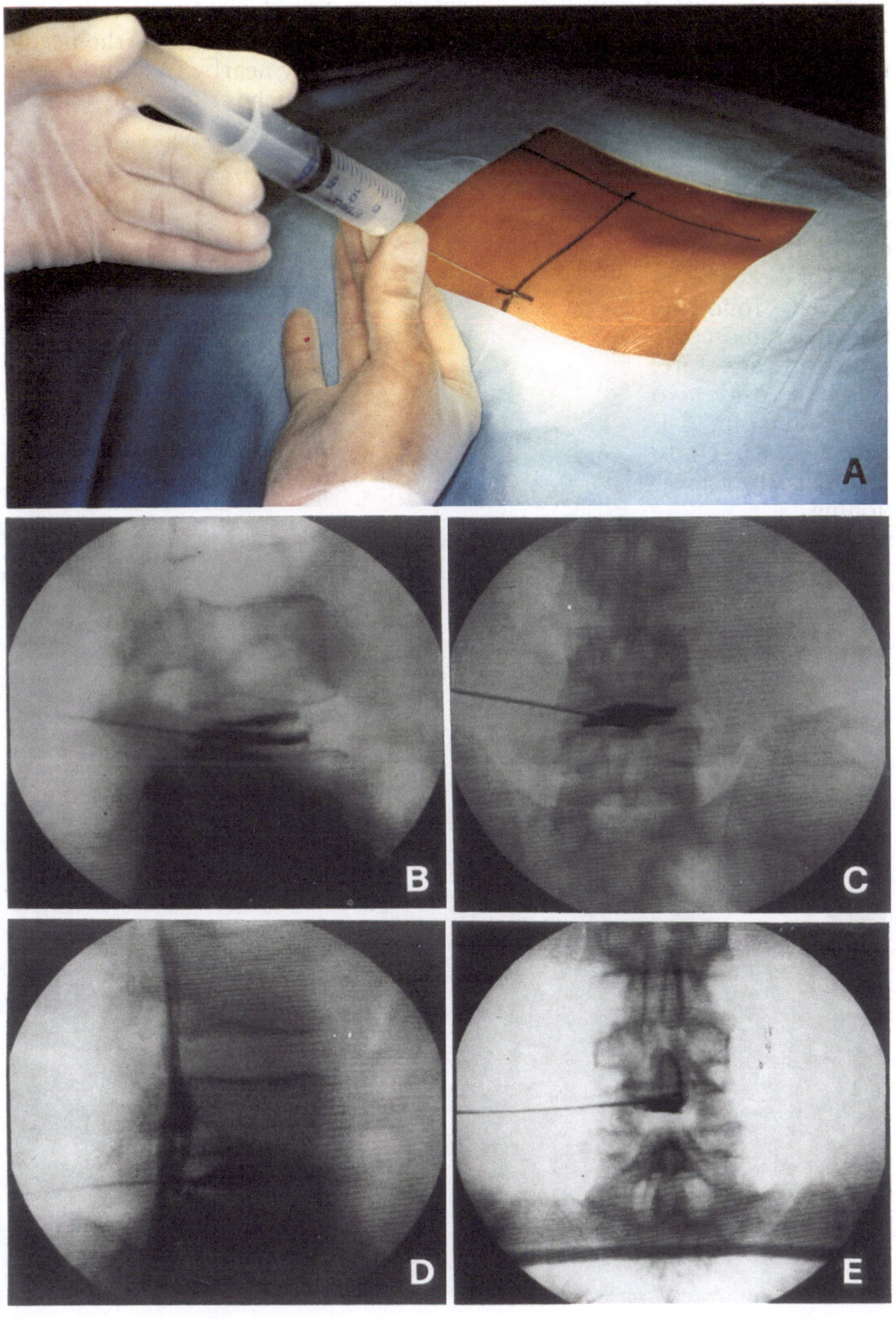

When the indication is confirmed, a skin incision is made approximately 2 mm in length in the area corresponding to the insertion site of the needle used for discography or in a site which is extremely nearby (A), and this is penetrated using the wire-guide (B) in a direction which is rigorously parallel to the needle itself.

When the center of the intervertebral disc has been reached, and the needle used for discography removed, following the same radioscopic procedures as before, it is best to use two radiograms in A-P and L-L (C, D) to record correct positioning.

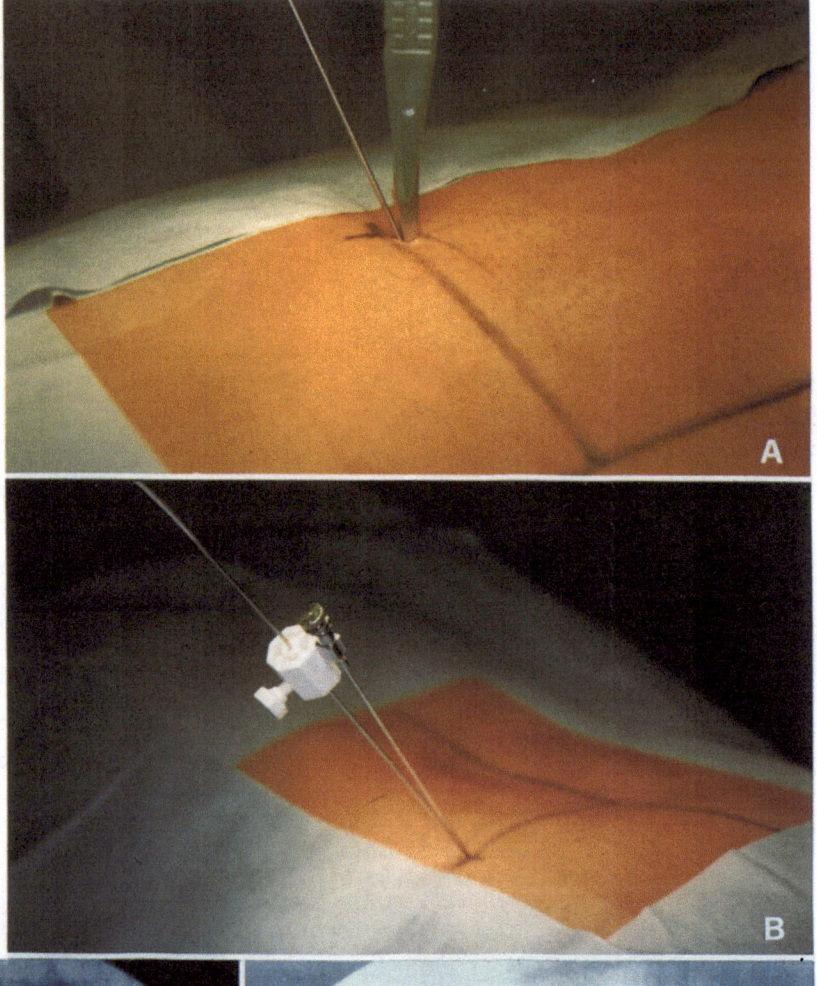

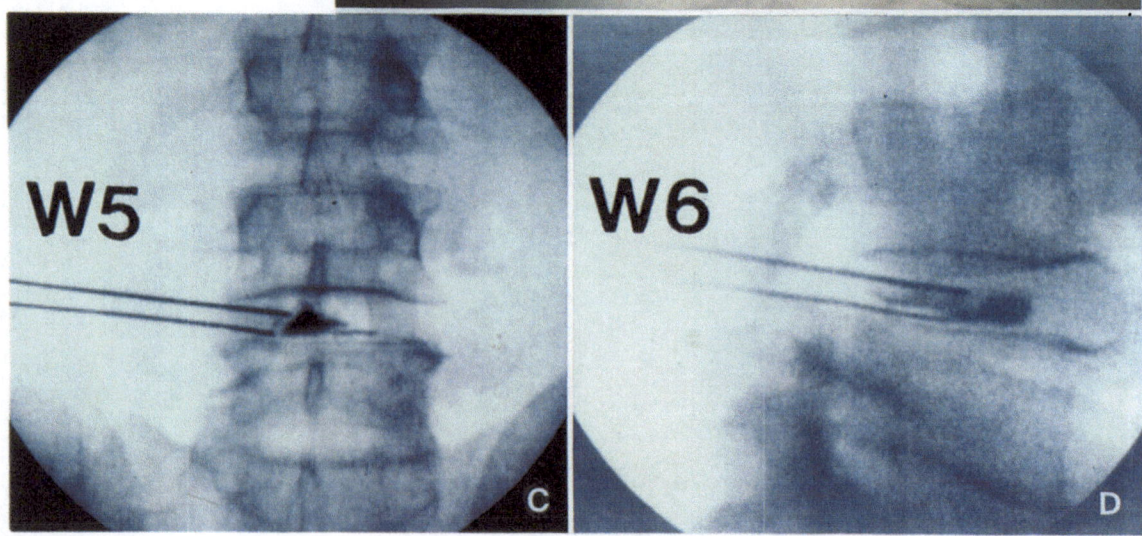

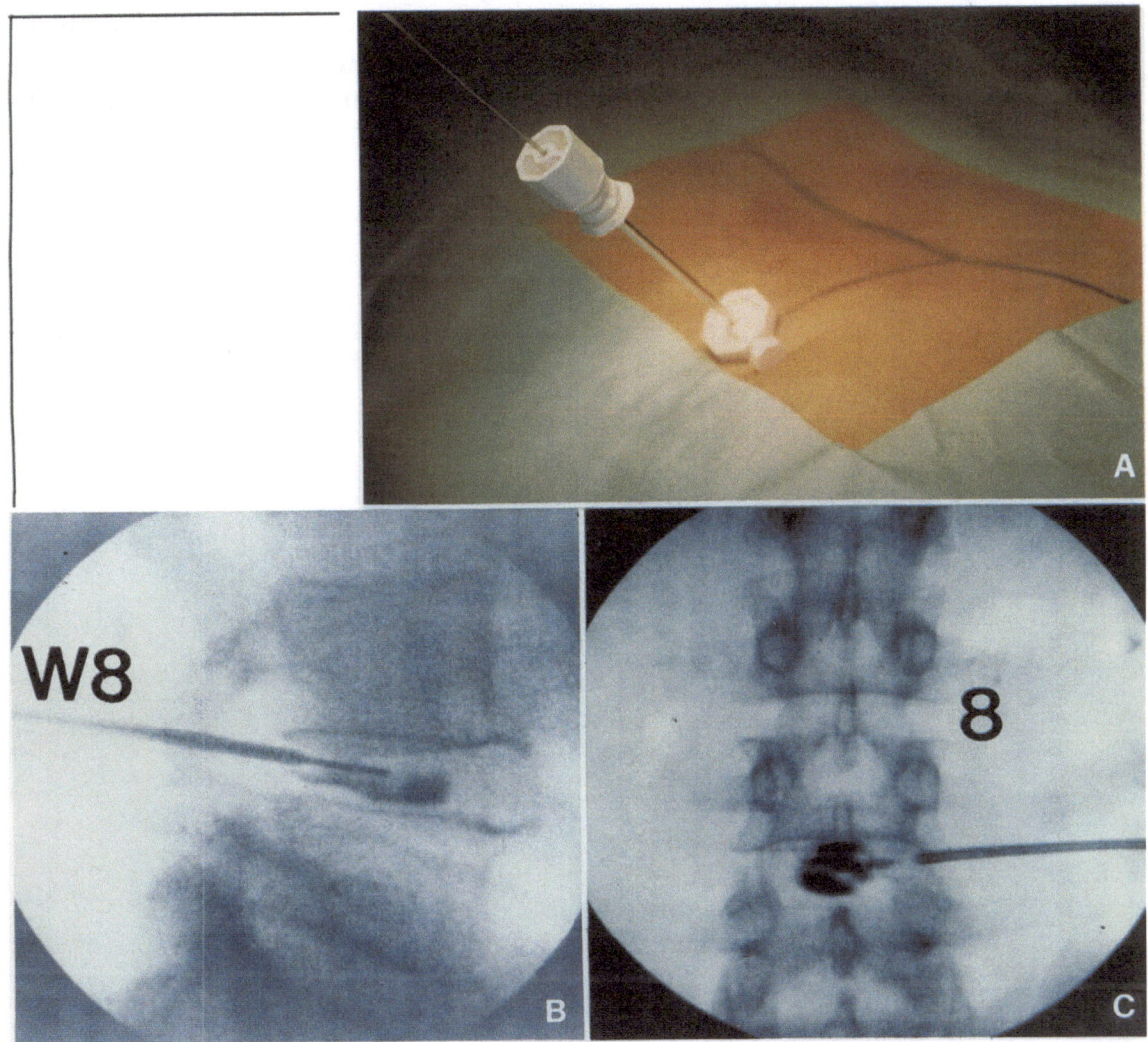

The needle used for discography is extracted and after the handle of the wire-guide has been removed, instrument 2 is inserted (sheath and dilator). The instrument is pushed until it moves up against the anulus fibrosus and allows the dilator to penetrate 2 mm: during this procedure the patient may complain of nerve root pain. Penetration of the dilator inside the anulus fibrosus seems to collapse easily, but the correct position will, at any rate, be confirmed by a radioscopic image in the two orthogonal projections (A-P and L-L), never relying on one of the images alone.

After the dilator has been extracted, leaving the sheath and the wire-guide in site, the anulus-breaker is inserted (A), which, thanks to its saw-toothed edge, allows us to make an 8 mm deep hole in the anulus fibrosus. This is obtained by making simultaneous rotation movements to push the instrument (B).

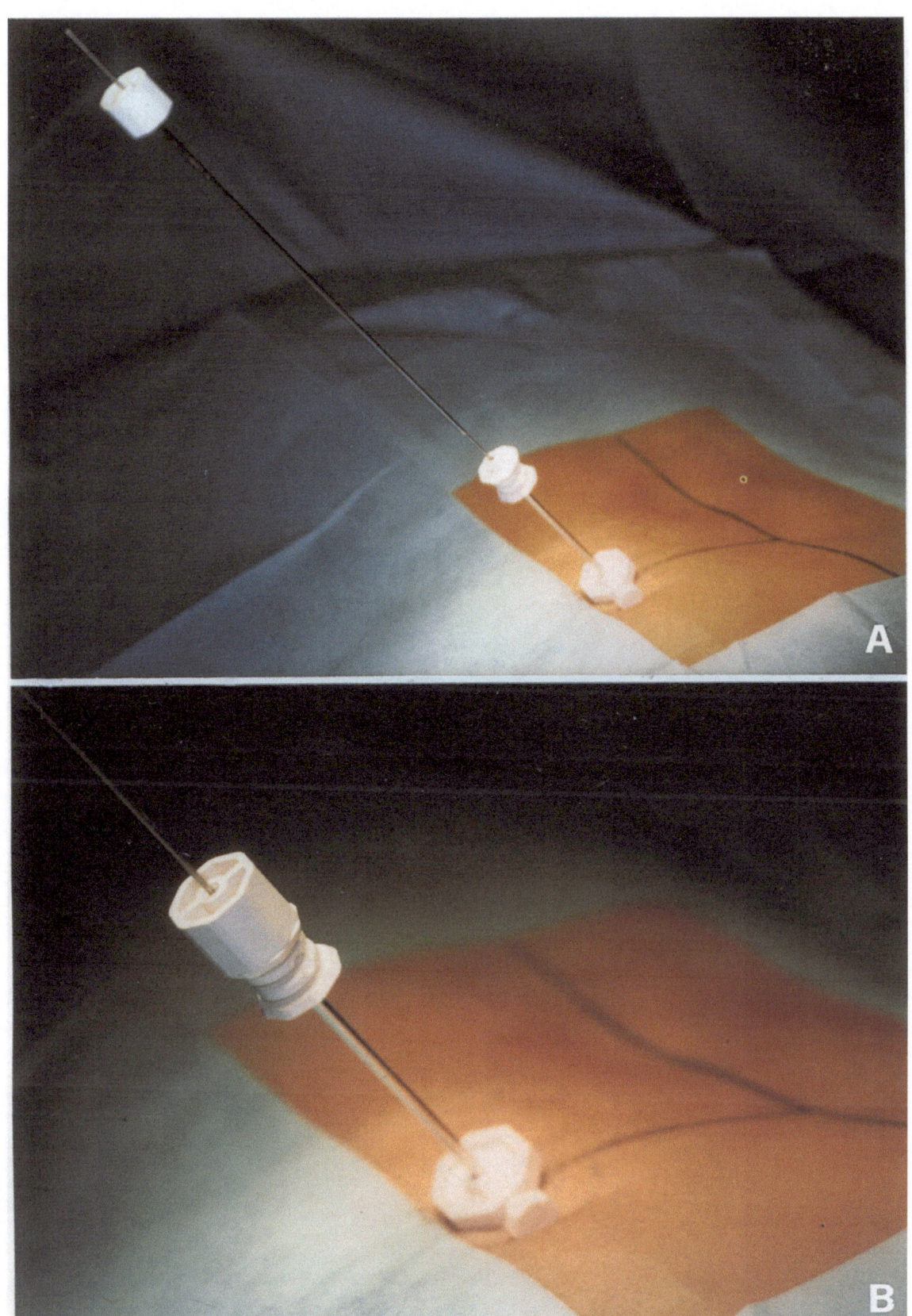

Keeping the sheath still, so that the arrest disc is stably in contact with the skin plane, the anulus-breaker and the wire-guide are extracted (A), and the nucleotome inserted (B).

The correct position of the instrument is checked under radioscopic monitoring (C, D).

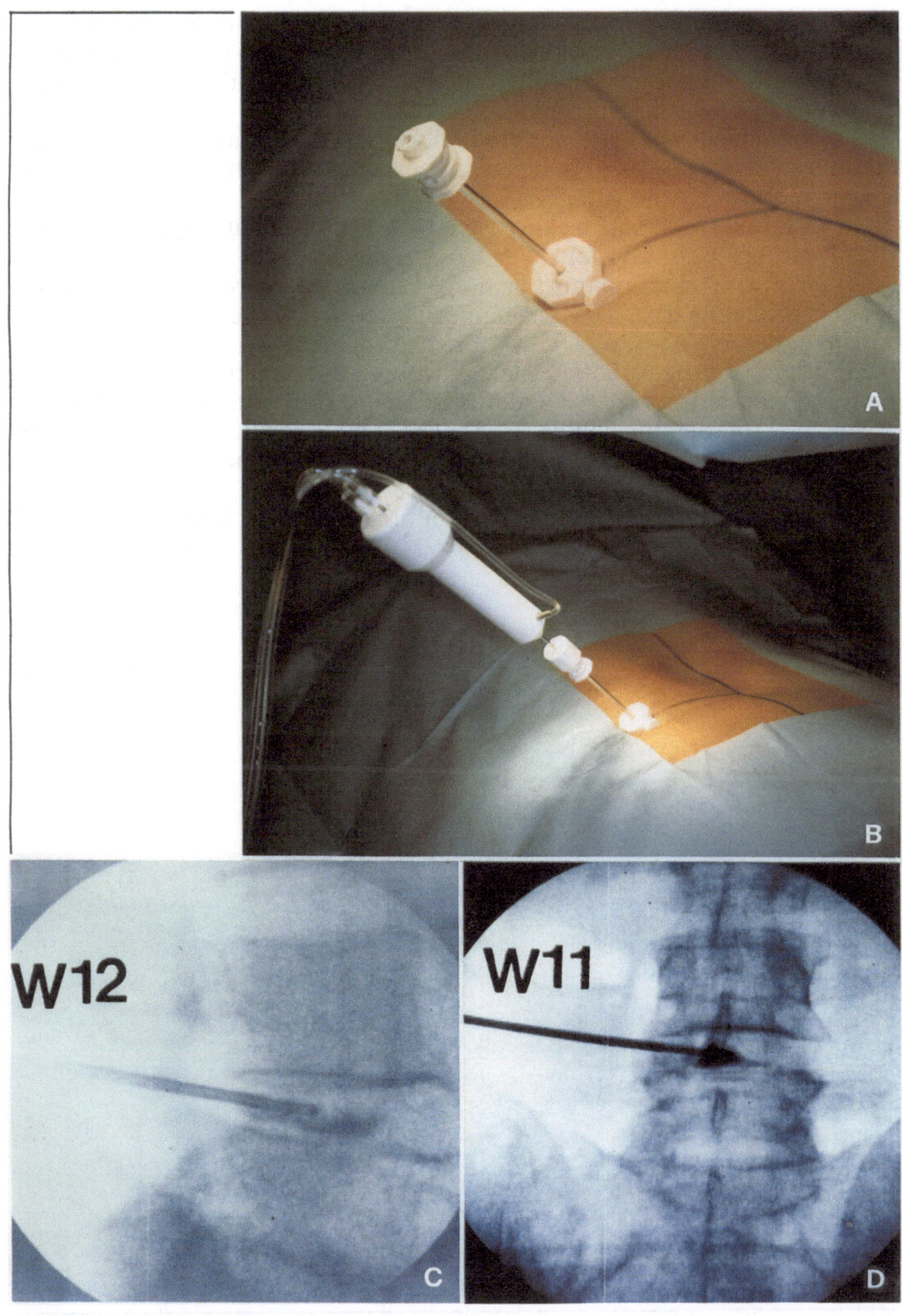

The nucleotome is now activated, using the pedal, and discectomy is initiated; this must be carried out making full use of the instrumentation:

1) first, it is important to begin with high frequency cutting thus producing a space within which to maneuver;

2) the frequency of cutting is gradually reduced, thus allowing more time for aspiration as opposed to fragmentation, so that small chips of disc material are pulled towards the cutter;

3) lavage phases should be alternated with aspiration-cutting phases (every 10' of cutting, 1' of lavage);

4) the instrumentation must be moved so as to explore as much space as possible inside the disc. This is obtained by retracting the nucleotome or by moving it deeper (A, B, C, D); as aforementioned, it has a 3 cm excursion;

5) it must not be forgotten that by varying the directions in the various sites, the loop-hole of the nucleotome is lateral, so it must be appropriately oriented by rotating the handle (E, F). The spatial position of the loop-hole may be imagined by referring to the lavage fluid tube handle, which is on the same side.

During the entire procedure the skin arrest must be kept still.

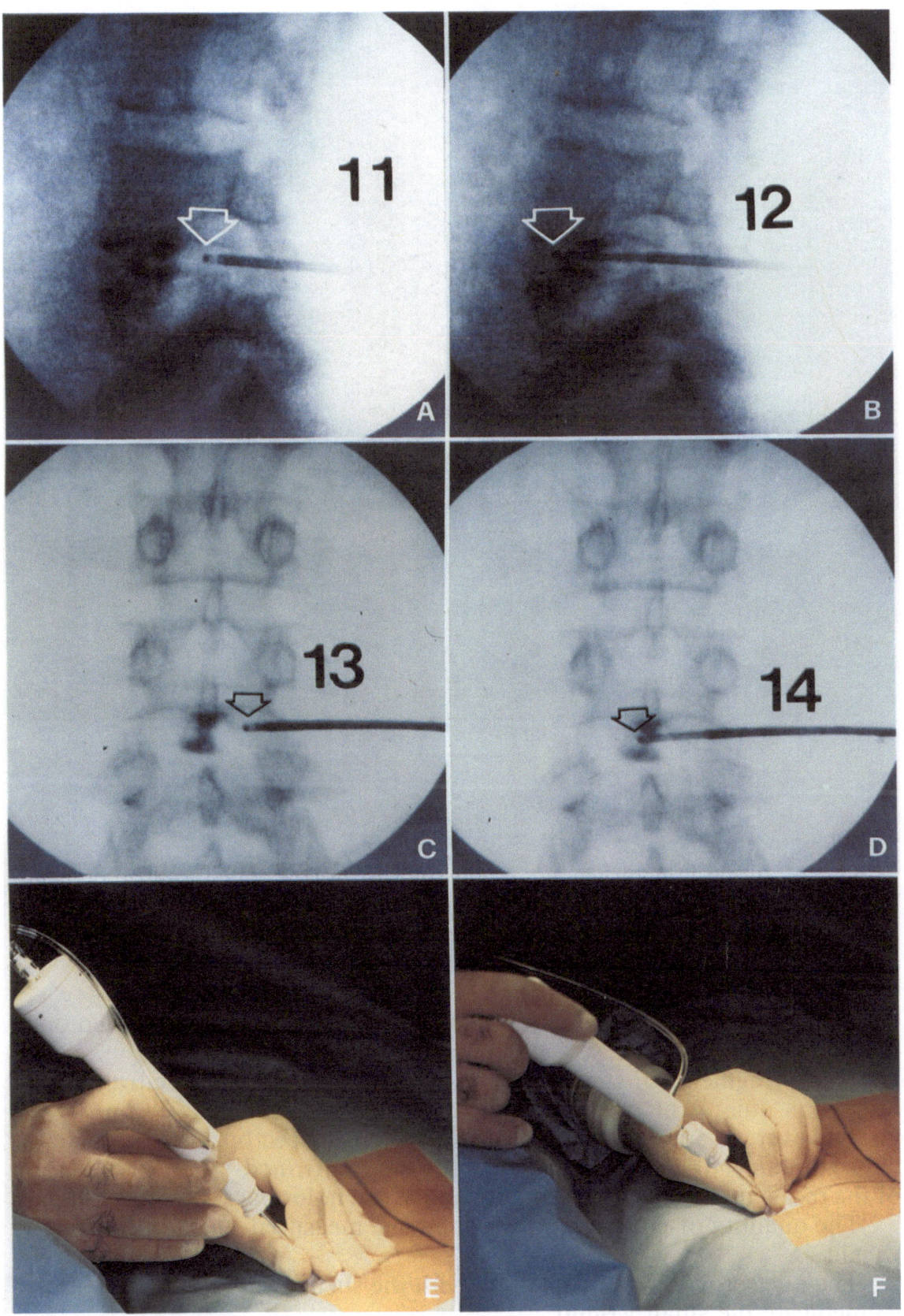

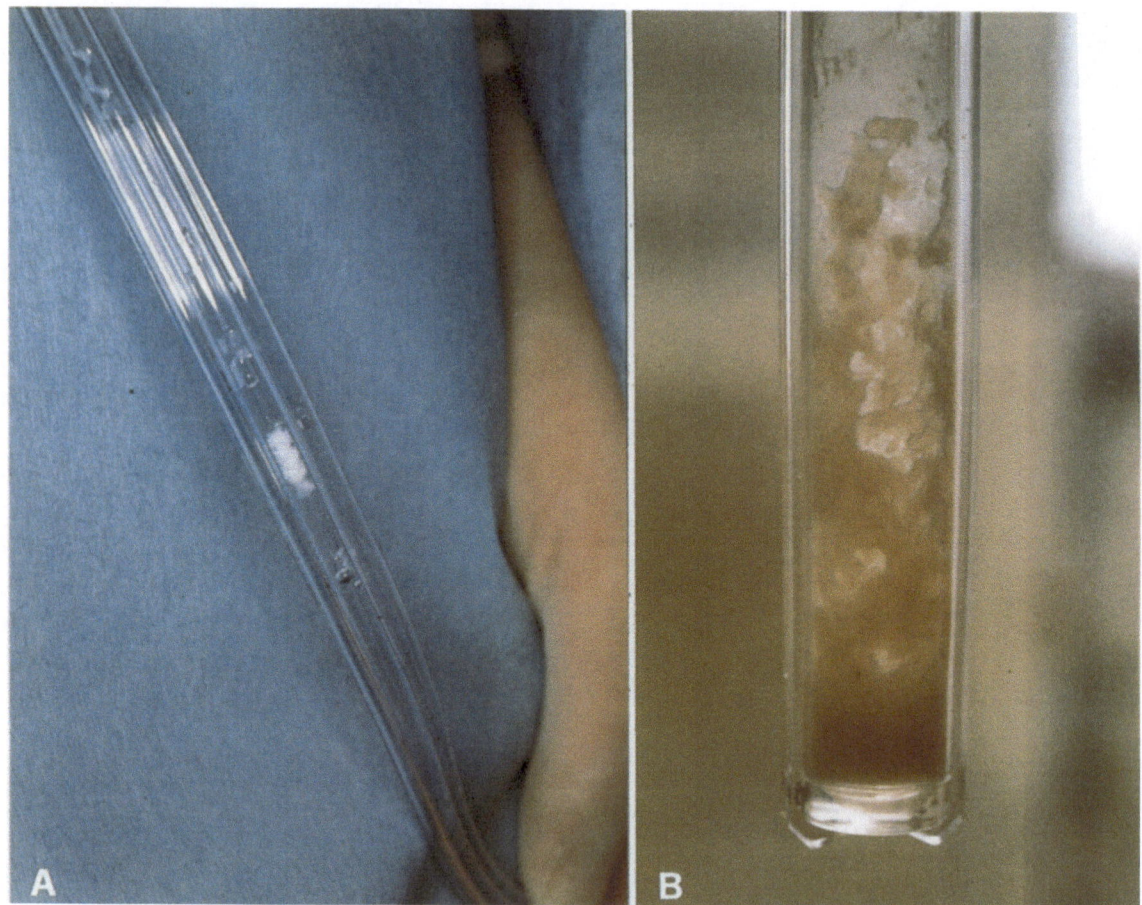

During surgery the movement of the nucleotome may be monitored visually, by observing the chips of disc tissue in the drainage tube (A), mixed with lavage fluid, constituted by an isotonic saline solution, under negative aspiration pressure ranging from 575 to 620 mmHg.

The lavage fluid must always be clear.

As the nucleus is removed, emptiness must be felt around the nucleotome, the movements of which are easier and more ample.

When fragments of the disc tissue are no longer seen in the transparent aspiration union, the operation has ended.

The average amount of time to affirm that discectomy has occurred is approximately 40-45 minutes; this is further confirmed by an examination of the recipient having a filtering test-tube which holds back the disc chips (B).

The quantity of material removed may be measured in terms of size and weight.

The nucleotome is then extracted with the sheath, and a bandage is used to medicate the small wound.

Norms of hygiene and rehabilitation for the patient submitted to percutaneous discectomy

S. Broggi

During the first days postsurgery (3-4 days) the patient need not do any exercise, but he must remain in a so-called antalgic rest position in bed (A), and in this position he must *very slowly* flex his thighs in alternating fashion on the pelvis (B), *never more than* 50-60 movements in a day. Furthermore, a pillow between the patient's legs in lateral decubitus may be of use (C). Walking may be allowed for not more than 30-40 consecutive minutes, alternated with bed-rest.

A sitting position is *not recommended* (the patient may eat while standing), *nor should the patient use* a car.

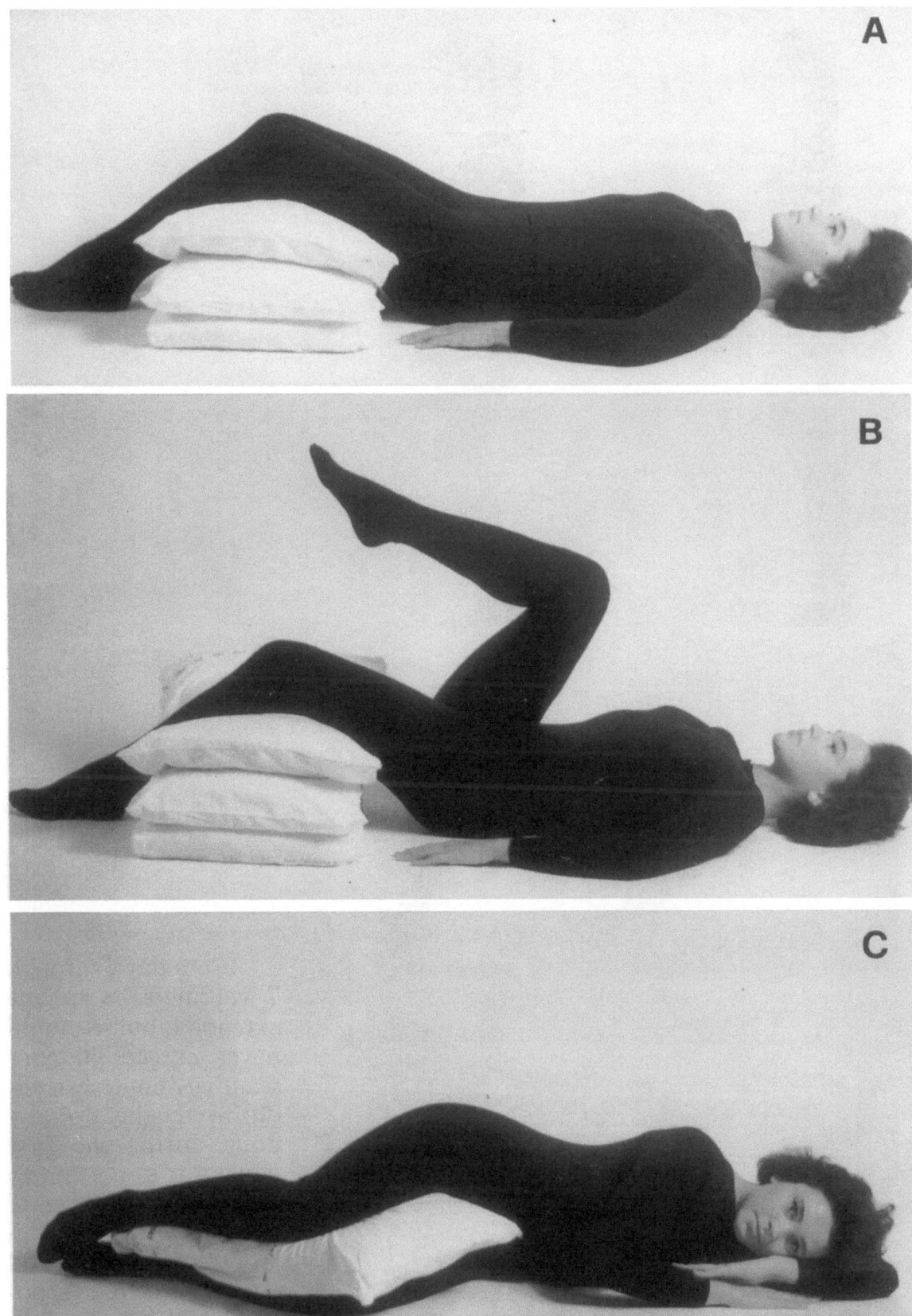

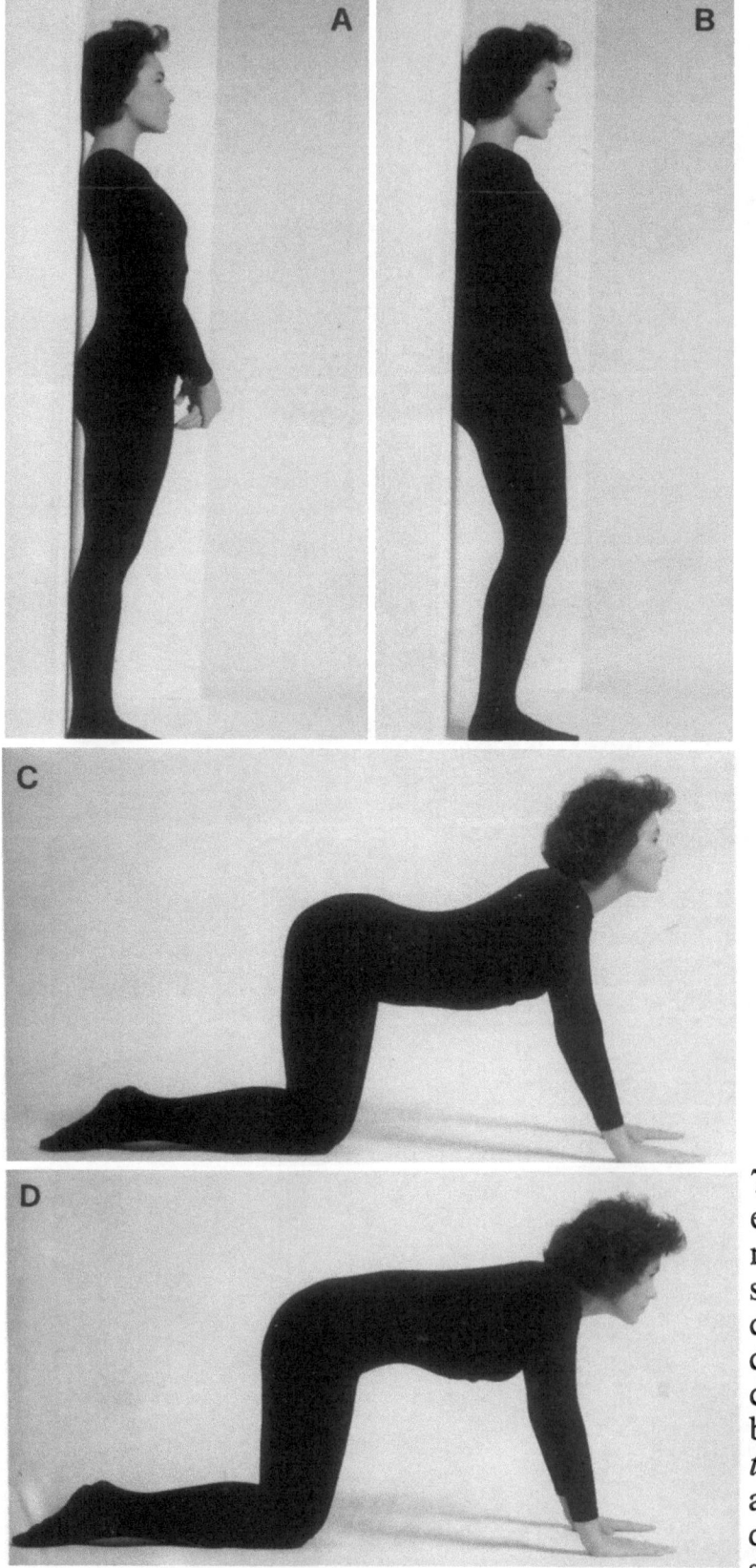

From day 4 through 7 walking time may be extended, but it should never exceed 60 consecutive minutes. In addition to the exercise done during the first days, it is important to begin exercise *to annul the lumbar lordosis* in an erect (A, B) and quadrupedic (C, D) position.

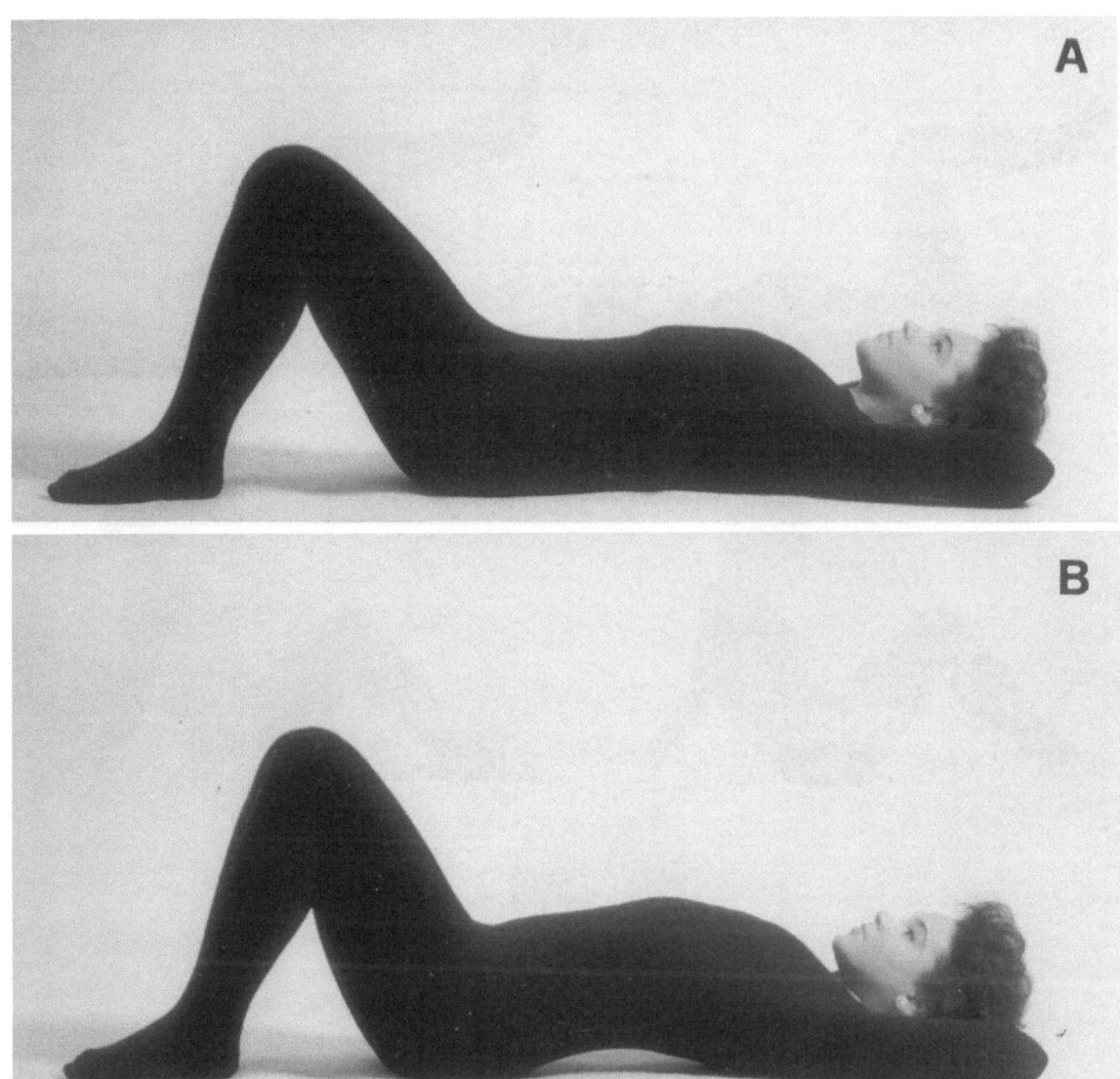

The exercise done to annul the lumbar lordosis should be done in a supine position on the floor (series of 10 movements every 2-3 hours in a day), in addition to those done in an erect position. The lumbar spine must be maintained *pressed* against the floor for 5-6 seconds (A) followed by relaxation for 20-30 seconds (B). All of the exercises must be done calmly, slowly, with no tearing or violence.

If there is a minimum amount of pain the patient should not interrupt exercising; however, if there is sciatic pain a physician should be consulted for pharmacological therapy (NSAIDS and myorelaxants), if necessary.

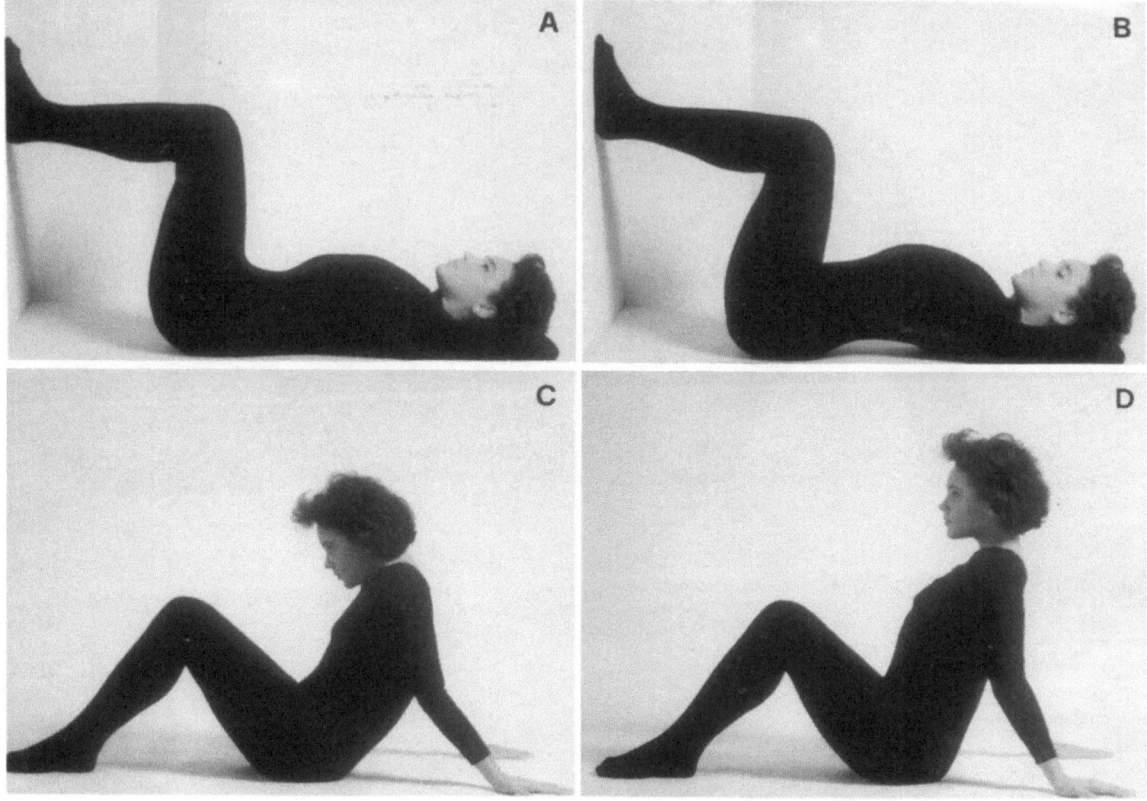

During the second week the patient may begin using the car, but only for short periods of time. *The patient must use a sitting position as little as possible.*

Exercises illustrated in (A, B) and (C, D) may be added, both for series of 10 movements not more than 3-4 times daily, and to alternate between periods of supine decubitus in bed and antalgic rest positions.

Now that walking is done for one hour or more, it is best to use a cloth brace, obviously to be removed while the patient is in bed.

Sexual activity may be resumed, with caution; in particular, positions may be varied with the partner's help, as long as pain is not re-awakened.

It is important that the patient know that mild lumbar pain is paraphysiological, and thus should cause no worry.

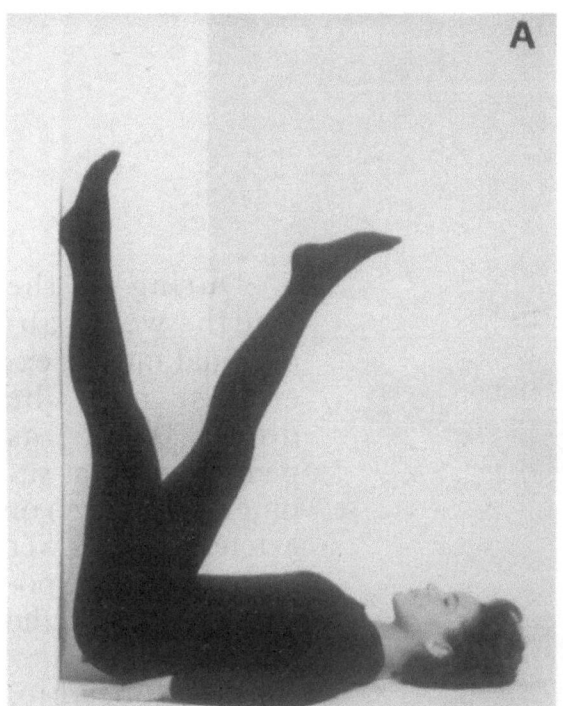

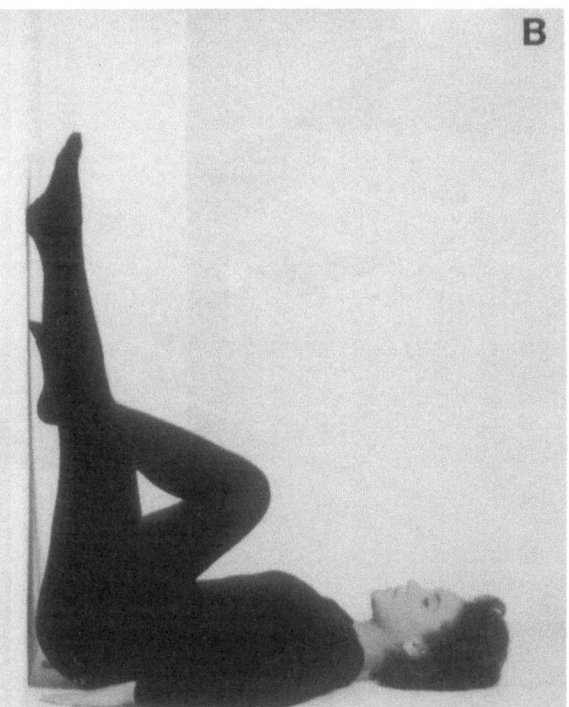

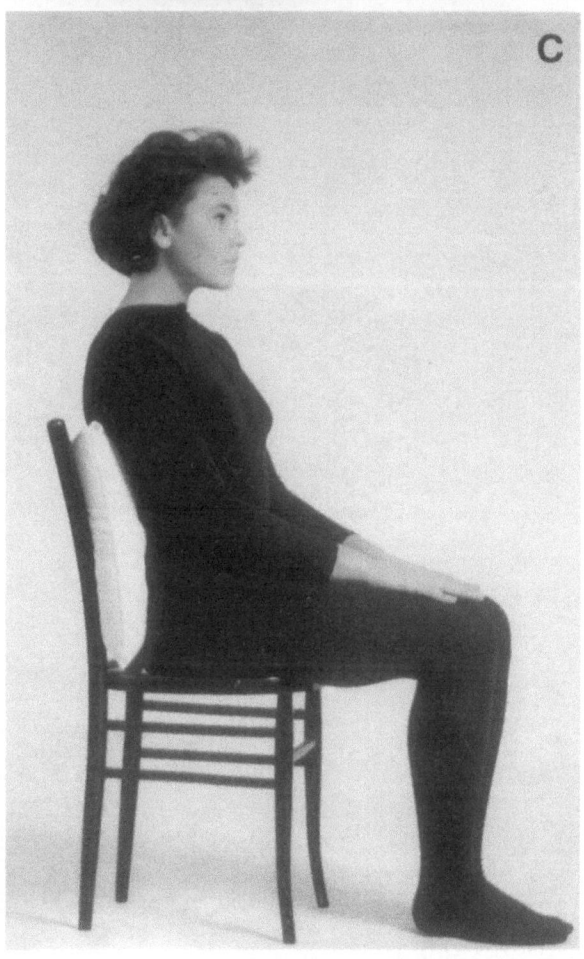

During the third week exercises (A) and (B) may be done; these are the most dangerous as they may re-awaken sciatic pain: if this should occur, they must be interrupted and resumed after a week.

When possible, it is advisable to begin a swimming program. At this point the patient may walk or hold an erect station for 2-3 hours consecutively.

Continue to avoid the sitting position for long periods of time, or at least, be sure to use a pillow against the back of the chair (C). Work may be resumed if sedentary, and if it allows for the patient to alternate a sitting position with a standing one, and if the work location is near home.

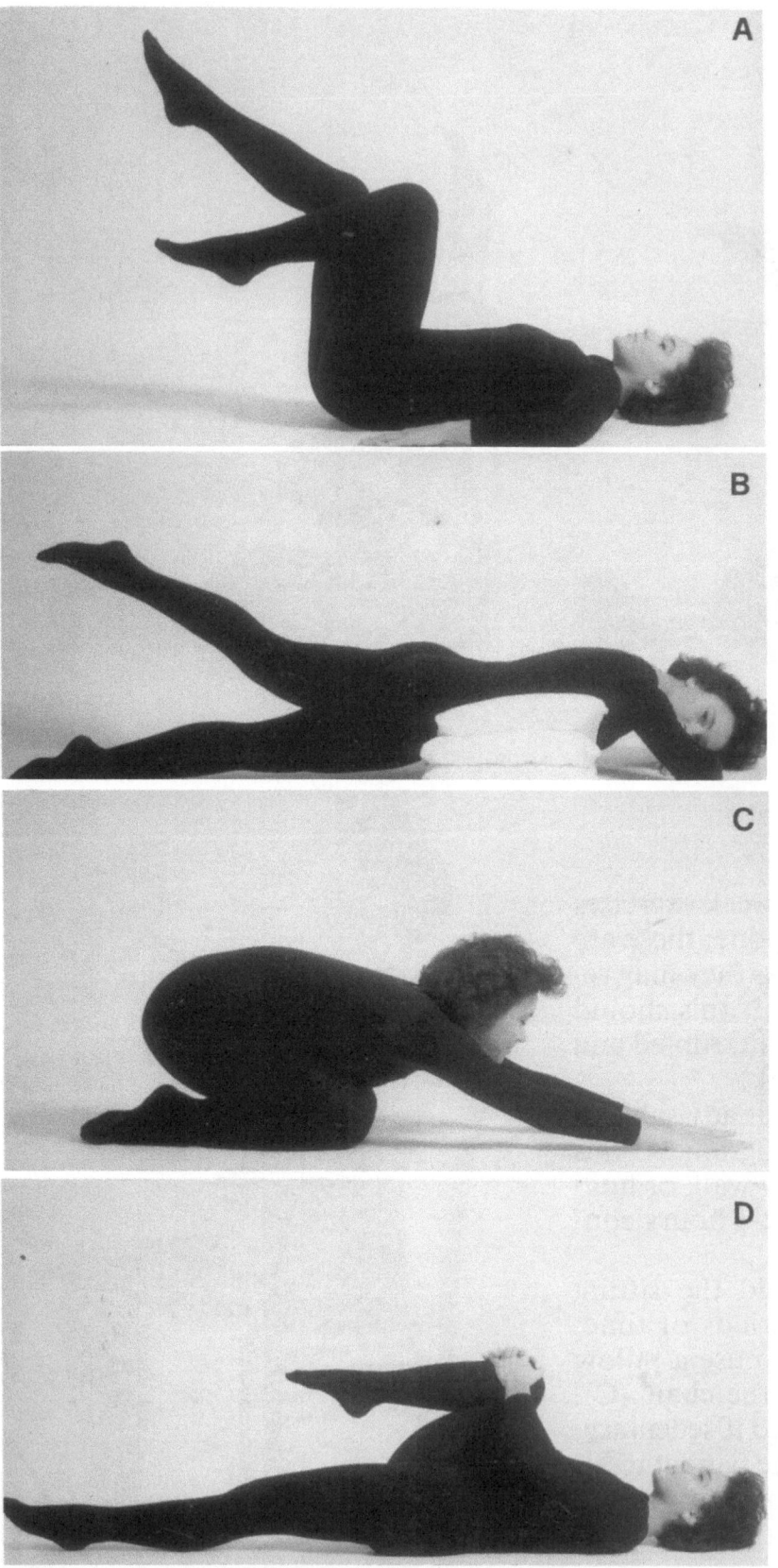

During the fourth week abdominal muscle exercises may be done, such as pedalling in a supine position (A) or extending the lower limbs in a prone position, reducing the lordosis (B).

If possible, swimming should be intensified.

Work in an office may without a doubt be resumed, as long as the patient may get up and walk frequently.

The car should not be used for trips longer than 100 km.

Stretching exercises are advised (C, D). Heavy work activity (bricklayer, truck-driver, etc.) cannot be resumed prior to 2 months, and only after monitoring by a physician.

After this period of time, competitive or amateur sports activity may be resumed.

Criteria for an evaluation of the results of percutaneous discectomy

N. Ruggieri

The literature reports numerous methods used to evaluate the results obtained after the treatment of spine pathology.

Nonetheless, in terms of a reading of the results of percutaneous discectomy, specific reference must be made to an evaluation of patients affected with lumbar sciatic pain syndromes and to the progression of the anomaly after treatment.

As we were able to specify in the previous chapters, in fact, the indication for use of the method, limited to those patients who have lumbar and nerve roots symptoms, appears to be essential; this is so not only in terms of well-known problems related to indication, but also for the sake of a future comparison between several homogeneous case series again with regard to indication.

Here reported are four classifications used to evaluate lumbar sciatic pain in reference to what may best identify the results of percutaneous discectomy:

— MacNab classification (1971), for laminectomy and based on the pain-activity binomial;

— Cabot classification (1977), originally aimed at evaluating laminectomy, taking into consideration activity and clinical data (pain, nerve root deficit, Lasègue), as well as the subjective opinion of the patient;

— Benoist classification (1982), used for postchemonucleolysis evaluation, which takes into consideration activity and symptoms, both lumbar and peripheral;

— Onik classification (1987) used by the inventor of the method precisely to evaluate percutaneous discectomy, which distinguishes between success and failure based on 5 criteria, of which 4 clinical-functional and 1 subjective.

MACNAB CLASSIFICATION (1971)

Excellent	No pain. Activity not restricted.
Good	Occasional pain in back or leg enough to interfere with normal work or leisure time activities.
Fair	Improvement in functional ability, but compromised by intermittent pain enough to reduce or modify work or leisure time activities.
Poor	No improvement; need for further surgery.

CABOT CLASSIFICATION (1977)

CLASS	I	II	III	IV
PARAMETERS	EXCELLENT	GOOD	FAIR	POOR
a) subjective improvement of patient	90-100%	70-90%	50%	0%
b) resumption of work activity	Yes (same job)	Yes (caution)	No (Only sedentary)	No
c) residual pain	—	+	+ +	+ + +
d) peripheral neurological deficit	—	—	—	+
e) Lasègue sign	>80 degrees	80-60 degrees	60-45 degrees	<45 degrees

BENOIST CLASSIFICATION (1982)

Very good	— No sciatica — Lumbar pain negligible or none — No neurological sequelae (except reflexed) — Normal activity
Good	— Fair residual sciatica — Moderate lumbar pain with stress — Partial limitation of activity
Poor	— Failure; further surgery required — Sciatic pain unchanged or worsened — Complete limitation of activity — Fair improvement with need for further treatment

ONIK CLASSIFICATION (1987)

CRITERIA USED TO DEFINE SUCCESS IN TREATMENT

1) Further surgery not required.
2) Irradiated pain improved a fair amount or totally.
3) Preoperative functional state of patient improved after surgery.
4) The patient no longer needs to take analgesics for sciatic pain.
5) Both the patient and the surgeon are satisfied with immediate results.

Failure is constituted by the absence of all 5 points.

Comments
A. Solini

Percutaneous discectomy according to the Onik method is not a difficult method, it makes use of simple instrumentation, but has rather restricted indications.

As previously stated, it is a method used to remove the intervertebral disc by percutaneous access and with closed surgery, and its main feature is the smaller diameter of the probe, the task of which is to fragment and aspire the small chips of pulpy nucleus.

This fact is probably positive because of the minor risk of discitic infection (described to occur in various percentages with all methods of percutaneous discectomy) and because of the small hole in the anulus which closes spontaneously after the probe is removed.

Some French authors who have recently used the Onik instrumentation system, report that there is less frequency of so-called 5th day syndrome. This involves acute lumbar pain, which is resolved in a few weeks of therapy with myorelaxants and anti-inflammatory drugs such as NSAIDs, often occuring after chemonucleolysis or percutaneous discectomy, the latter being carried out with instruments of larger diameter. According to some, this syndrome would be due to a retropsoic hematoma, in some cases revealed by magnetic resonance tomography, according to others by a settling of the segment of intervertebral movement, in particular, of the interapophysary joints.

For these and other reasons the Gary Onik method is being used more and more in Europe by various types of specialists: orthopaedists, neurosurgeons, and neuroradiologists. On our continent this method was first introduced in June 1987 and our group was probably the first to put it into practice. We believe that it constitutes a true act of surgery, and that it may only be performed in an operating room, the only location guaranteeing the required asepsis. One must be prepared to accept a certain number of failures (intraoperative discography revealing loss of contrast medium) and ready to propose the use of traditional surgery.

A patient may be submitted to percutaneous discectomy according to Onik if the following two basic requirements are met:

a) the parameters of the so-called Maroon and Onik protocol must be rigorously respected, and

b) the disc herniation must be contained, that is, the posterior longitudinal ligament and the posterior part of the anulus fibrosus must be whole, even if deformed.

In the previous pages we dealt with various aspects of the method, emphasizing indications and limits; I wish to express two concepts which I believe to be of importance and which are the product of my own experience:

1) to submit patients to this type of treatment who do not complain of lumbar and sciatic pain, with prevalence of the latter over the former, means altering the original protocol;

2) there is no preoperative means of establishing whether or not a disc herniation is contained.

Apart from any philosophy of imaging, intraoperative discography alone is capable of telling us whether or not a hernia is contained. Thus, we believe this to be an essential test, an integral part of the entire method, but one which, precisely because it is intraoperative, must be based on an accurate selection of the patients, and particularly in terms of a *clinical examination*. Let us recall, for example, that French colleagues never submit patients to chemonucleolysis or percutaneous discectomy if the patient has not observed a period of bed-rest for two to three weeks.

As for the technical aspects of discography, nothing more needs to be added to what is said in the specific chapter: however, I wish to emphasize once again the importance of performing a **true** nucleography, and not an anulography.

It may be interesting to note that according to some authors who perform discectomy (Roy-Camille and Schreiber), within certain limits, the **quantity** of disc tissue removed is not important, as there does not seem to be any relationship between the volume of herniary material removed and the clinical results. We consider the fact to be worthy of further study, even if it is based on a logical presupposition of the sufficiency of disc **distension** to obtain nerve root **decompression**.

Other considerations, which we have thought about, are also important.

An *evaluation of the results* is made based on different classification systems. During recent months, this method has been discussed at only a few meetings, and we have heard authors propose the MacNab, Benoist, or Cabot classification systems with relative indifference. Clearly, any comparison of the data, and particularly if long-term, cannot benefit from this. We use the Cabot classification system because we consider it to be the most suited and the most complete for a correct evaluation of the results. This system is not necessarily the best and we are willing to change it, should a *single* evaluation criterion be proposed, to be used by all those who perform percutaneous discectomy.

On the other hand, instrumental monitoring (computerized tomography, magnetic resonance tomography, etc.) cannot at present provide data which may be referred to the clinical results of discectomy: we recently heard Roy-Camille affirm that there is no relationship between the quality of the results and the postoperative radiological image and that, paradoxically, at times, poor results are characterized by a good radiological image. This, as well, needs to be changed in time. To this purpose we wish to clarify the fact that, in our opinion, the follow-ups obtained for these patients must be longer; just as the results of traditional herniectomy must be evaluated aftr many years, so a method which is just beginning to be used cannot be judged as having obtained good or excellent results one or two months postsurgery.

In our first 40 cases, followed-up after 3 to 6 months, using the Cabot classification system, we observed a decrease in good results, from 29% to 25%, and an increase in fair results, from 16% to 20%. This observation, which we believe to have made in a rigorous manner, makes us think.

The results obtained by us and by other authors may be defined comforting: this means that the method must be applied without superficial enthusiasm, and in particular, that these results must be submitted to a more prolonged evaluation in time.

Appendix

J.A. TAYLOR ANXIETY QUESTIONNAIRE

Name of patient	Age	Sex	Profession	Clinical record n.

Diagnosis

Therapy

Date onset treatment	Posology

INSTRUCTIONS

Carefully read each definition and underline either «true» if the conditions indicated are in fact true, or «false» if there is no symptom.

EVALUATION: capital letter anxiety response (1 point)

1) I don't get tired early	true	FALSE	
2) I often feel nauseated	TRUE	false	
3) I don't think that I am more nervous than others	true	FALSE	
4) I have very few headaches	true	FALSE	
5) I am very tense when I work	TRUE	false	
6) I can't concentrate my thoughts on one thing	TRUE	false	
7) I worry about money and business	TRUE	false	
8) I notice that my hand often trembles when I try to do something	TRUE	false	
9) I don't blush more than others	true	FALSE	
10) I have diarrhoea more than once a month	TRUE	false	
11) I don't worry too much about possible disasters	TRUE	false	
12) I never blush	true	FALSE	
13) I often worry about blushing	TRUE	false	
14) I often have nightmares	TRUE	false	
15) My hands and feet are usually warm	true	FALSE	
16) I often perspire even on cold days	TRUE	false	
17) When I am in an embarrassing situation I perspire, and this bothers me	TRUE	false	
18) I hardly ever hear my heart beat, and I am rarely short of breath	true	FALSE	
19) I am always hungry	TRUE	false	
20) I am hardly ever constipated	true	FALSE	
21) I have many gastric disorders	TRUE	false	

22) I have had very bothersome periods of insomnia	TRUE	false	
23) I sleep fitfully	TRUE	false	
24) I often dream about myself	TRUE	false	
25) I am often embarrassed	TRUE	false	
26) I am more sensitive than others	TRUE	false	
27) I often worry about things	TRUE	false	
28) I would like to be happy like other people	TRUE	false	
29) I am usually calm and never get upset	true	FALSE	
30) I cry easily	TRUE	false	
31) I am always anxious about something or someone	TRUE	false	
32) I am more or less happy	true	FALSE	
33) I become nervous if I am asked to wait	TRUE	false	
34) I get so nervous that I can't sit still for a long time	TRUE	false	
35) At times I'm so excited that I can't sleep	TRUE	false	
36) At times I have the feeling that my problems are so many that I can't overcome them	TRUE	false	
37) I must admit that at times I worry about things that don't really exist	TRUE	false	
38) I am not very apprehensive as compared to my friends	true	FALSE	
39) I am frightened by things or people that I know can't hurt me	TRUE	false	
40) Sometimes I feel useless	TRUE	false	
41) I have difficulty concentrating on a task or on work	TRUE	false	
42) I am exceptionally self-critical	TRUE	false	
43) I make things hard for myself	TRUE	false	
44) I am a very tense person	TRUE	false	
45) For me life is usually tiring	TRUE	false	
46) Sometimes I think I am good for nothing	TRUE	false	
47) I never have faith in myself	TRUE	false	
48) At times I feel like I'm coming apart	TRUE	false	
49) I get tense when there is a crisis or difficulty	TRUE	false	
50) I have extreme faith in myself	true	FALSE	
		Total score	
Therapy ended on	Experimenter		

B.W. ROCKLIFF SELF-RATING QUESTIONNAIRE FOR DEPRESSION (SRQ-D)*

Name of patient		Age	Sex	Profession		Clinical record n.

Diagnosis

_____

_____

_____

Therapy

_____

_____

Date onset treatment	Posology

Mark an answer for the questions	rarely or never	some-times	quite often	nearly always	total score
1) Do you feel tired for no reason?	0	1	2	3	
2) Does noise irritate you?**					
3) Do you feel demoralized or sad?	0	1	2	3	
4) Do you like music?**					
5) Do you feel particularly sad in the morning?	0	1	2	3	
6) Do you get involved in arguments?**					
7) Do you feel like crying?	0	1	2	3	
8) Do you have migraine headaches?**					
9) Do you wake up early and have difficulty falling back to sleep?	0	1	2	3	
10) Do you often have accidents or hurt yourself?**					
11) Do you have loss of appetite?	0	1	2	3	
12) Do you find watching television fun?**					
13) Do you feel that your life is empty?	0	1	2	3	
14) Do you have difficulty thinking clearly?	0	1	2	3	
15) Do you avoid people and social contacts?	0	1	2	3	
16) Do you feel that others would be better off if you were dead?	0	1	2	3	
17) Do you feel that you no longer appreciate things that you once did?	0	1	2	3	
18) Do you feel like you're not worth much as a person?	0	1	2	3	

How to use scale
a score of 3: person normal
a score of 18: patient more or less depressed
** Questions monitoring ability to answer (do not evaluate)

Comments:

_____

_____

_____

Therapy ended on	Experimenter

* (Self-Rating Questionnaire for Depression)

S. CROWN AND A.H. CRISP SELF-RATING QUESTIONNAIRE FOR PSYCHONEUROTIC PATIENTS (MHQ)*

Name of patient	Age	Sex	Profession	Clinical record n.

Diagnosis
_____
_____
_____

Therapy
_____
_____

Date onset treatment	Posology

INSTRUCTIONS

The questions refer to your feelings or actions. They are all simple. Mark the box corresponding to the answer which you feel is applicable to your case. Don't spend too much time on any one question.

1) DO YOU FEEL DISTURBED WITHOUT REASON?

☐ yes   ☐ no

2   0

2) DO YOU FEEL UNREASONABLY AFRAID IN A CLOSED SPACE SUCH AS A SHOP, AN ELEVATOR, ETC.?

☐ often   ☐ sometimes   ☐ never

2   1   0

3) DO PEOPLE EVER SAY THAT YOU ARE TOO SCRUPULOUS?

☐ no   ☐ yes

0   2

4) ARE YOU AFRAID OF HEIGHTS OR OF SUFFOCATING?

☐ never   ☐ often   ☐ sometimes

0   2   1

5) CAN YOU THINK AS QUICKLY AS USUAL?

☐ yes   ☐ no

0   2

6) ARE YOUR OPINIONS EASILY INFLUENCED?

☐ yes   ☐ no

2   0

7) DO YOU FEEL LIKE YOU ARE FAINTING?

☐ often   ☐ sometimes   ☐ never

2   1   0

* (Middlesex Hospital Questionnaire)

(continues)

8) ARE YOU AFRAID THAT YOU MAY HAVE AN INCURABLE DISEASE?		
☐ never	☐ sometimes	☐ often
0	1	2

9) DO YOU BELIEVE THAT PURITY IS CLOSE TO A SENSE OF RELIGION?	
☐ yes	☐ no
2	0

10) DO YOU OFTEN FEEL ILL AFTER DIGESTING POORLY?	
☐ yes	☐ no
2	0

11) DO YOU THINK THAT LIFE IS TOO TIRING AND DIFFICULT?		
☐ at times	☐ often	☐ never
1	2	0

12) HAVE YOU EVER IN YOUR LIFE FOUND PLEASURE IN REACTING?	
☐ yes	☐ no
2	0

13) DO YOU FEEL ANXIOUS AND RESTLESS?		
☐ often	☐ sometimes	☐ never
2	1	0

14) DO YOU FEEL MORE RELAXED AT HOME?		
☐ without a doubt	☐ sometimes	☐ not particularly
2	1	0

15) DO YOU CONSTANTLY HAVE SILLY THOUGHTS?		
☐ often	☐ sometimes	☐ never
2	1	0

(continues)

16) DO YOU SOMETIMES FEEL LIKE YOU ARE ITCHING OR HAVE INSECT BITES ON YOUR BODY, LEGS, ARMS?

☐ hardly ever	☐ often	☐ never
1	2	0

17) DO YOU REGRET THE PAST?

☐ yes	☐ no
2	0

18) DO YOU NORMALLY CONSIDER YOURSELF TO BE A VERY EMOTIONAL PERSON?

☐ yes	☐ no
2	0

19) DO YOU OFTEN PANIC?

☐ no	☐ yes
0	2

20) DO YOU FEEL ILL-AT-EASE ON A BUS OR ON A SUBWAY EVEN IF NOT CROWDED?

☐ very much so	☐ a little	☐ not at all
2	1	0

21) DO YOU FEEL HAPPY WHEN YOU WORK?

☐ yes	☐ no
2	0

22) HAS YOUR APPETITE DECREASED LATELY?

☐ no	☐ yes
0	2

23) DO YOU WAKE UP UNUSUALLY EARLY?

☐ yes	☐ no
2	0

(continues)

24) ARE YOU HAPPY TO BE AT THE CENTER OF ATTENTION?

☐ no   ☐ yes

0   2

25) DO YOU THINK YOU ARE AN ANXIOUS PERSON?

☐ very much so   ☐ quite so   ☐ not at all

2   1   0

26) DO YOU HATE TO GO OUT ALONE?

☐ yes   ☐ no

2   0

27) ARE YOU A PERFECTIONIST?

☐ no   ☐ yes

0   2

28) DO YOU FEEL TIRED OR EXHAUSTED WITHOUT REASON?

☐ often   ☐ sometimes   ☐ never

2   1   0

29) DO YOU HAVE LONG PERIODS OF SADNESS?

☐ never   ☐ often   ☐ sometimes

0   2   1

30) DO YOU TAKE ADVANTAGE OF THE CIRCUMSTANCES?

☐ never   ☐ sometimes   ☐ often

0   1   2

31) DO YOU AT TIMES FEEL TERRIBLY TENSE INSIDE?

☐ yes   ☐ no

2   0

(continues)

32) DO YOU WORRY MORE THAN NECESSARY IF A RELATIVE IS LATE COMING HOME?

☐ no   ☐ yes

0   2

33) DO YOU FEEL THE NEED TO VERIFY BEYOND EVERY LIMIT THE THINGS THAT YOU DO?

☐ yes   ☐ no

2   0

34) AT PRESENT DO YOU SLEEP WELL?

☐ no   ☐ yes

2   0

35) DO YOU HAVE TO MAKE A BIG EFFORT TO DEAL WITH A CRISIS OR WITH A PROBLEM?

☐ very much so   ☐ sometimes   ☐ not more than usual

2   1   0

36) DO YOU SPEND A LOT OF MONEY ON CLOTHING?

☐ yes   ☐ no

2   0

37) HAVE YOU EVER HAD THE FEELING THAT YOU WERE FALLING APART?

☐ yes   ☐ no

2   0

38) ARE YOU AFRAID OF HEIGHTS?

☐ very much so   ☐ quite so   ☐ not at all

2   1   0

39) ARE YOU ANNOYED IF YOUR NORMAL ROUTINE IS DISTURBED?

☐ considerably   ☐ a little   ☐ not at all

2   1   0

(continues)

40) DO YOU OFTEN PERSPIRE EXCESSIVELY OR FEEL YOU HEART BEAT RACE?		
☐ no	☐ yes	
0	2	

41) DO YOU NEED TO CRY?		
☐ often	☐ sometimes	☐ never
2	1	0

42) DO YOU LIKE DRAMATIC SITUATIONS?		
☐ yes	☐ no	
2	0	

43) DO YOU HAVE NIGHTMARES THAT BOTHER YOU WHEN YOU MAKE UP?		
☐ never	☐ sometimes	☐ often
0	1	2

44) DO YOU PANIC IN A CROWD?		
☐ always	☐ sometimes	☐ never
2	1	0

45) DO YOU FEEL UNREASONABLE AND ILL-AT-EASE FOR THINGS WHICH HAVE NO REAL IMPORTANCE?		
☐ never	☐ often	☐ sometimes
0	2	1

46) HAS YOUR INTEREST IN SEX CHANGED?		
☐ less	☐ the same or more	
2	0	

47) HAVE YOU LOST YOUR ABILITY TO FEEL PLEASURE AT THE THOUGHT OF OTHERS?		
☐ no	☐ yes	
0	2	

48) DO YOU FEEL THAT YOU ARE ACTING AT TIMES?		
☐ yes	☐ no	
2	0	

(continues)

Part for the experimenter to fill in.

SUBDIVISION OF SCORE INTO SUBGROUPS

A N X I E T Y

Question n.	1	7	13	19	25	31	37	43	TOTAL
Score									

P H O B I A S

Question n.	2	8	14	20	26	32	38	44	TOTAL
Score									

O B S E S S I O N S

Question n.	3	9	15	21	27	33	39	45	TOTAL
Score									

S O M A T I C   D I S O R D E R S

Question n.	4	10	16	22	28	34	40	46	TOTAL
Score									

D E P R E S S I O N

Question n.	5	11	17	23	29	35	41	47	TOTAL
Score									

H Y S T E R I A

Question n.	6	12	18	24	30	36	42	48	TOTAL
Score									

Therapy ended on   Experimenter

References

ARMSTRONG J. R.: The causes of unsatisfactory results from the operative treatment of lumbar disc lesions. *J. Bone and Joint Surg.*, **33B**, 31-35,1951.

BENOIST M.: Traitement de sciatiques discales par chimionucléolyse (120 observations). *Rev. Chir. Orthop.*, **68**, 4, 261-267, 1982.

BENOIST M., DEBURGE A., BUSSON J.: La chimionucléolyse dans le traitement des sciatiques par hernie discale. *Presse Méd.*, **13**, 733-736,1984.

BENOIST M., ROCOLLE J., BUSSON J., POLACK Y., DEBURGE A.: *Résultat de la chimionucléolyse - Enquête européenne (discase R)*. In: *La Chimionucléolyse*, 125-138. Labo Armour Montagu, Levallois Perret, 1984.

BERGER P.E., ATKINSON D., WILSON W.J., WILTSE L.: High-resolution surface coil MRI of the spine: Normal and pathological anatomy. *Radiographics*, **6**, 573,1986.

BERSI G.: *La chemionucleolisi nell'ernia discale lombare*. Libreria Cortina, Torino, 1980.

BIANCHI M., RUFFONI R.: L'osteoartrite intersomatica vertebrale secondaria a laminectomia per ernia discale. *Arch. Ortop.*, **75**, 1024,1962.

BOBEST M.: H Nuclear Magnetic Resonance study of intervertebral discs. A preliminary report. *Spine*, **11**, 7, 709-711, 1986.

BOMBELLI R.: Il disco intervertebrale, sua patologia e visualizzazione mediante discografia. *Arch. Ortop.*, **66**, 705, 1953.

BONNEVILLE J.F.: *Focus on chemonucleolysis*. Springer Verlag, Berlin-Heidelberg, 1986.

BONOLA A., BEDESCHI P.: Acquisizioni anatomo-cliniche e miglioramenti tecnici nella chirurgia delle lombosciatalgie. *Arch. Putti*, **21**, 76-90, 1966.

BOUILLET R.: Complications of discal hernia therapy. Comparative study regarding surgical therapy and nucleolysis by chymopapain. *Acta Orthop. Belg.*, **49-suppl.**, 48-77, 1983.

BRADFORD D.S., OEGEMA T.R., COOPER K.M.: Chymopapain, chemonucleolysis and nucleus pulposus regeneration. *J.*

Bone and Joint Surg., **65A**, 1220, 1983.

BROWN M.D.: Diagnosis of pain syndromes of the spine. *Orthop. Clin. North Am.*, **6**, 233-248, 1975.

BROWN M.D., PANJABI M., LINDAHL S. *et al.*: *Measurement of disc degeneration by simultaneous volume and pressure recordings during discography*. Read before the International Society for the Study of the Lumbar Spine, Toronto, 1982.

CABOT J.R.: *Cirugia del dolor lumbosacro*. Valladolid, 1977.

CALVÉ J., GALLAND M.: The intervertebral nucleus pulposus: its anatomy, its physiology, its pathology. *J. Bone Joint Surg.*, **12**, 555, 1930.

DEBURGE A., BENOIST M., BOYER D.: The diagnosis of disc sequestration. *Spine*, **9**, 496-499, 1984.

DEBURGE A., BENOIST M., ROCOLLE J.: La chirurgie dans le échecs de la nucléolyse des hernies discales lombaires. *Rev. Chir. Orthop.*, **70**, 637-641, 1984.

DELITALA F., BONOLA A.: *Ernia del disco e sciatica vertebrale*. Cappelli, Bologna, 1949.

DE MARCHI E., BELGRANO M.: I risultati lontani del trattamento chirurgico dell'ernia del disco intervertebrale. *Chir. Org. Mov.*, **36**, 57-65, 1951.

DEL TORTO U.: La via laterale e il discografo di Marino-Zuco per la visualizzazione dei dischi intervertebrali. *Atti 42° Congr. SIOT*, 339, 1957.

DEL TORTO U.: Contributo allo studio della fisiopatologia del disco intervertebrale attraverso le immagini discografiche. *Ortop. Traumat. App. Mot.*, **3**, 1961.

DYCK P.: Paraplegia following chemonucleolysis. A case report and discussion of neurotoxicity. *Spine*, **10**, 4, 359-362, 1985.

EDEIKEN J., PITT N.J.: The radiologic diagnosis of disc disease. *Orthop. Clin. North Am.*, **71**, 405, 1978.

EDWARDS W. *et al.*: CT discography: prognostic value in selection of patients for chemonucleolysis. *Spine*, **12**, 792, 1987.

EPSTEIN J.A., EPSTEIN B.S., LAVINE L.: The effect of anatomic variations in the lumbar vertebrae and spinal canal on Cauda equina and nerve root syndromes. *Am. J. Roentgenology*, **91**, 1055-1063, 1964.

ERLACHER P.R.: Nucleography. *J. Bone Joint Surg.*, **34B**, 204, 1952.

FINESCHI G.F.: *Patologia e clinica dell'ernia posteriore del disco intervertebrale.* Edizioni Scientifiche Istituto Ortopedico Toscano, 1955.

FINESCHI G.F., PALANDRI C.: Rilievi statistici su 1020 casi di ernia del disco lombare. *Arch. Putti*, **5**, 301, 1954.

FIROOZNIA H., BENJAMIN V., KRICHEFF I. et al.: CT of lumbar spine disk herniation: Correlation with surgical findings. *AJNR*, **5**, 91, 1984.

FRIEDMAN: Percutaneous discectomy: An alternative to chemonucleolysis? *Neurosurg.*, **13**, 5, 542, 1983.

GADO M., PATEL J., HODGES F.J.: Lateral disk herniation into the lumbar intervertebral foramen: differential diagnosis. *Am. J. Neuroradiol.*, **4**, 598-606, 1983.

GANDOLFI M.: *Storia della sciatica.* Cappelli, Bologna, 1965.

GANDOLFI M.: *Clinica e terapia delle protrusioni posteriori dei dischi intervertebrali lombari.* Aulo Gaggi, Bologna, 1966.

GANDOLFI M., JUCOPILLA N., TOMASSO A.: *La T.A.C. - Discografia lombare.* Atti 12° Congr. SIRC, II, 1459. Monduzzi, Bologna, 1986.

GANDOLFI M., JUCOPILLA N., TOMASSO A.: *La chemionucleolisi, la discectomia al microscopio e la chirurgia tradizionale nel trattamento della sindrome sciatalgica.* Atti 12° Congr. SIRC, II, 1475, Monduzzi, Bologna, 1986.

GARVIN P.J., JENNINGS R.B., STERN I.J.: Enzymatic digestion of the nucleus pulposus: a review of experimental studies with chymopapain. *Orthop. Clin. North Am.*, **8**, 27, 1977.

HAUGHTON V.M., ELDEVIK P.O., MAGNAES B. et al.: A prospective comparison of CT and myelography in the diagnosis of herniated lumbar disk. *Radiology*, **142**, 103, 1982.

HELFET A.J., GRUBEL LEE D.M.: *Patologia della colonna vertebrale.* Verduci, Roma, 1979.

HICKEY D.S.: Analysis of magnetic resonance images from normal and degenerate lumbar intervertebral discs. *Spine*, **11**, 7, 702-708, 1986.

HICKEY D.S., HUKINS D.W.L.: Relations between the structure of the anulus fibrosus and the function and failure of the intervertebral disc. *Spine*, **5**, 2, 106, 1980.

HIJIKATA S.: Perkutane Nukleotomie — neue Behandlung der Diskushernie. *J. Toden Hosp.*, **5**, 39, 1975.

HIJIKATA S., YAMAGISHI M., NAKAYAMA T., OOMORI K.: Percutaneous discectomy: a new treatment method for lumbar disc herniation. *J. Toden Hosp.*, **5**, 5, 1975.

HOFFMAN G.S.: Spinal arachnoiditis. What is the clinical spectrum? *Spine*, **8**, 5, 538-540, 1983.

HOPPER K., SHERMAN J., KUETHKE J. et al.: The retrorenal colon in the supine and prone patient. *Radiology*, **162**, 443, 1987.

HUDGINS W.R.: Computer-aided diagnosis of lumbar disc herniation. *Spine*, **8**, 6, 604-615, 1983.

INOUE S., WATANABE T., HIROSE A., TANAKA T., MATSUI N., SAEGUSA O., SHO E.: Anterior diskectomy and interbody fusion for lumbar disc herniation: a review of 350 cases. *Clin. Orthop.*, **183**, 22, 1984.

JACCHIA G.E.: Casistica, risultati e cause di insuccessi di ernie discali operate. *Atti 65° Congr. SIOT*, 1980.

JACKSON R.K.: The long-term effects of wide laminectomy for disc excision. A review of 130 patients. *J. Bone Joint Surg.*, **53B**, 609-616, 1971.

KAHANOVITZ N.: The effect of discography on the canine intervertebral disc. *Spine*, **11**, 1, 26-27, 1986.

KAMBIN P., GELLMAN H.: Percutaneous lateral discectomy of the lumbar spine. A preliminary report. *Clin. Orthop.*, **174**, 127, 1983.

KAMBIN P., SAMPSON S.: Posterolateral percutaneous suction-excision of herniated intervertebral discs. *Clin. Orthop.*, **207**, 37, 1986.

KEHR P., LANG G., PATERNOTTE H.,

TRENSZ T.H.: Comment essayer techniquement d'éviter les èches dans la chirurgie des hernies discales. *Rev. Chir. Orthop.*, **68**, 4, 254-257, 1982.

KHALIFA P., BOISSONAS A., GIRAUDET J.S., SERENI D., CREMER G.A., LAROCHE C.: Syndrome de la queue de cheval au décours d'une nucléolyse. *Rev. Rhum.*, **55**, 311, 1984.

KICUCHI S., HASUE M.: Anatomic and clinical studies of radicular symptoms. *Spine*, **9**, 1, 1984.

KIRKALDY-WILLIS W.H.: The relationship of structural pathology to the nerve root. *Spine*, **9**, 1, 49-52, 1984.

LAWLESS G.F., SELBY D., HINNANT D., McCOY C.E.: Reduction of postoperative pain parameters by presurgical relaxation instructions for spinal pain patients. *Spine*, **10**, 650, 1985.

LINDHOLM T.S., PILKKANEN P.: Discitis following removal of intervertebral disc. *Spine*, **7**, 618-622, 1982.

LOEW F., CASPAR W.: *Surgical approach to lumbar disc herniation. (The micro-approach to the lumbar disc prolapse operation). Advances and technical standards in neurosurgery*, 5. Springer Verlag, Berlin - Heidelberg - New York, 1978.

LOUIS R.: *Chirurgie du rachis.* Springer-Verlag, Berlin-Heidelberg, New York, 1982.

MACKINNON S.E., HUDSON A.R., DELLON A.L., KLINE D.G., HUNTER D.A.: Peripheral nerve injury by chymopapain injection. *J. Neurosurg.*, **61**, 1-8, 1984.

MACNAB I.: Chemonucleolysis. *Clin. Neurosurg.*, **20**, 183-192, 1973.

MACNAB I.: Negative disc exploration. An analysis of the causes of nerve-root involvement in sixty-eight patients. *J. Bone Joint Surg.*, **53A**, 891-903, 1971.

MAROON J.C., HOLST R.A., OSGOOD C.P.: Chymopapain in the treatment of ruptured lumbar discs; preliminary experience in 48 patients. *J. Neurol. Neurosurg. Psychiat.*, **39**, 508-513, 1976.

MAROON J.C., ONIK G.: Percutaneous automated discectomy. *J. Neurosurg.*, **66**, 143, 1987.

MILETTE P.C., MELANSON D.: Lumbar discography. *Radiology*, **163**, 828, 1987.

MODIC M.T., MASARIK T.J., PAUSHTER D.M.: MRI of the spine. *Radiol. Clin. North Am.*, **24**, 229, 1986.

MODIC M.T., PAVLICEK W., WEINSTEIN M.A. *et al.*: MRI of intervertebral disc disease: clinical and pulse sequence considerations. *Radiology*, **152**, 103, 1984.

MULAWKA S.M.: Chemonucleolysis. The relationship of the physical findings, discography and mielography to the clinical result. *Spine*, **11**, 4, 391-396, 1986.

NACHEMSON A., ELFSTRÖM G.: Intravital dynamic pressure measurements in lumbar discs. A study of common movements, maneuvres and exercises. *Scand. J. Rehabil. Med.* (suppl.), **1**, 1970.

NACHEMSON A., LEWINE T., MAROUDAS A., FREEMAN R.: In vitro diffusion of dye through the end plates and annulus fibrosus of human lumbar intervertebral disc. *Acta Orthop. Scand.*, **41**, 589-607, 1970.

NACHEMSON A., MORRIS J.M.: In vivo measurements of intradiscal pressure: discometry, a method for the determination of pressure in the lower lumbar discs. *J. Bone Joint Surg.*, **46A**, 1077-1092, 1964.

NAYLOR A.: The late results of laminectomy for lumbar disc prolapse. A review after ten to twenty-five years. *J. Bone Joint Surg.*, **56B**, 17-28, 1974.

NAZARIAN S.: Anatomical basis of intervertebral disc puncture with chemonucleolysis. *Anat. Clin.*, **7**, 23-32, 1985.

NGO F., BOUMPHREY M.D., MODIC M.: *The basis of Magnetic Resonance Imaging of intervertebral disc.* FOSA, S. Francisco, 1987.

NORDBY E.J., LUCAS G.L.: A comparative analysis of lumbar disk disease treated by laminectomy or chemonucleolysis. *Clin. Orthop.*, **90**, 119, 1973.

OLSSON S.E.: Observations concerning disc fenestration in dogs. *Acta Orthop. Scand.*, **20**, 349, 1950.

ONIK G., HELMS C.A.: *Automated percutaneous lumbar discectomy.* Radiology Research and Education Foundation. S. Francisco, 1988.

ONIK G., HELMS C.A., GINSBERG L., HOA-

GLUND F.T., MORRIS J.: Percutaneous lumbar diskectomy using a new aspiration probe: porcine and cadaver model. *Radiology*, **155**, 251-252, 1985.

ONIK G., HELMS C.A., GINSBERG L., HOAGLUND F.T., MORRIS J.: Percutaneous lumbar diskectomy using a new aspiration probe. *Am. J. Neurorad.*, **6**, 290-293, 1985.

ONIK G., MAROON J.C., HELMS C.A., SCHWEIGEL J., MOONEY V., KAANOVITZ N., MORRIS J., McCULLOCH J.A., REICHER M.: Automated percutaneous diskectomy: initial patient experience. *Radiology*, **162**, 129-132, 1987.

PARK W.M., McCALL I.W., O'BRIEN J.P., WEBB J.K.: Fissuring of the posterior annulus fibrosus in the lumbar spine. *British J. Radiol.*, **52**, 382-387, 1979.

PAUSHTER D.M., MODIC M.T., MASARYK T.J.: MRI of the spine: applications and limitations. *Radiol. Clin. North Am.*, **23**, 551, 1985.

PECH P., HAUGHTON V.M.: Lumbar intervertebral disk: correlative MR and anatomic study. *Radiology*, **156**, 699, 1985.

POSTACCHINI F., LAMI R., FACCHINI M.: *Risultati a confronto tra chimonucleolisi e intervento chirurgico in pazienti con ernia discale lombare*. Atti 2° Congr. SIRC, II, 1465-1467. Monduzzi, Bologna, 1986.

RASKIN S.P., KEATING J.W.: Recognition of lumbar disc disease: comparison of mielography and CT. *Am. J. Roentgenology*, **139**, 349, 1982.

RAVICHANDRIAN G., MULLHOLLAND R.C.: Chymopapain chemonucleolysis. *Spine*, **5**, 380-384, 1980.

ROMY M.: Chemonucleolysis technique: new oblique approach requires no measurements. *J. Neurol. Orthop. Med. Surg.*, **6**, 1, 47, 1985.

SALVI V.: La tomografia assiale computerizzata nella diagnosi di ernia discale lombare. *Giornale It. Ortop. Traumat.*, **11**, 47-54, 1985.

SALVI V.: *La chimonucleolisi nel trattamento dell'ernia del disco lombare*. Minerva Medica, Torino, 1985.

SALVI V., BOUX E.: La chimonucleolisi con chimopapaina nell'ernia discale lombare. (Considerazioni sui primi cento casi con controllo da tre mesi a tre anni). *Min. Ortop.*, **37**, 123-132, 1986.

SCAGLIETTI O., FINESCHI G.F.: Ernie discali post-foraminali nella colonna lombare. *Arch. Putti*, **17**, 556-565, 1962.

SCHNEIDERMAN G., FLANNAGAN B., KINGSTON S., THOMAS J., DILLING W.H., WATKINS R.G.: Magnetic Resonance Imaging in the diagnosis of disc degeneration: correlation with discography. *Spine*, **12**, 276-281, 1987.

SCHREIBER A., SUEZAWA Y.: Trandiscoscopy percutaneous nucleotomy in disk herniation. *Orthop. Review*, **XV**, 1, 75-78, 1986.

SCHUIERER G.: *NMR imaging of the spine and spinal canal*. Atti 1° Simposio Europeo su «Lombalgia e Lombosciatalgia». Cortina, Torino, 1982.

SENEGAS J., LAVIGNOLLE B.: Dégénérescence discale, syndrome des facettes et rhizolyse lombaire per-cutanée. *Entretiens Médecine et Rééducation Simon*, 7, 313-324, 1984.

SHAPIRO R.: Current status of lumbar discography. *Radiology*, **159**, 815, 1986.

SHAPTER A.E.: Current status of lumbar discography. *Radiology*, **161**, 853, 1986.

SIMEONE F.A., ROTHMAN R.H.: Clinical usefulness of CT scanning in the diagnosis and treatment of lumbar spine disease. *Radiol. Clin. North Am.*, **21**, 197, 1983.

SMITH L.: Enzyme dissolution of the nucleus pulposus in humans. *J.A.M.A.*, **187**, 137, 1964.

SMITH L., BROWN J.E.: Treatment of lumbar intervertebral disc lesions by direct injection of chymopapain. *J. Bone Joint Surg.*, **49B**, 502, 1967.

SMITH L., GARVIN P.J., JENNINGS R.B., GESLER R.M.: Enzyme dissolution of the nucleus pulposus. *Nature*, **198**, 1311, 1963.

SOLINI A., ORSINI G., PASCHERO B.: Nuclectomia percutanea lombare secondo Onik: indicazioni, principi tecnici, primi risultati. *Giornale It. Ortop. Traumat.*, **14**, 453-466, 1988.

SOLINI A. PASCHERO B., BROGGI S.: Importanza della valutazione psicoalgesimetrica nei pazienti cervicobrachialgici e lombosciatalgici. *Ortop. Traumat. Oggi*, **14**, 3, 243-249, 1984.

STRINGA G.: Reinterventi in sindromi radicolari lombari: indicazioni, tecnica, risultati. *Atti 65° Congr. SIOT*, 1980.

STRINGA G., MARCHETTI N.: Le ernie dei dischi lombari alti. *Atti 51° Congr. SIOT*, 1966.

SUEZAWA Y., JACOB H.A.C.: Percutaneous nucleotomy: an alternative to spinal surgery. *Arch. Orthop. Trauma Surg.*, **105**, 287-295, 1986.

SUEZAWA Y., RÜTTIMAN B.: Indikation Methodik und Ergebnisse der perkutanen Nukleotomie bei lumbaler Diskushernie. *Z. Orthop.*, **121**, 25-29, 1983.

TEPLICK J.G., HASKIN M.E.: CT and lumbar disc herniation. *Radiol. Clin North Am.*, **21**, 259, 1983.

VERBIEST H.: Pathomorphologic aspects of developmental lumbar stenosis. *Orthop. Clin. North Am.*, **6**, 117-196, 1975.

VERBIEST H.: *Neurogenic intermittent claudication. With special reference to stenosis of the lumbar vertebral canal.* Amsterdam-Oxford: North Holland, New York American Elsevier, 1976.

VLAHOVITCH B. *et al.*: Cinetique du produit de contraste en discographie lombaire. *Journée Montpellieraine d'Orthopedie*, 1978.

WHITE A.A., PANJABI M.M.: *Clinical biomechanics of the spine.* J.B. Lippincott Co., Philadelphia, 1978.

WILEY J.J., MacNAB I., WORTZMAN G.: Lumbar discography and its clinical applications. *Can. J. Surg.*, **11**, 280, 1968.

WILLIAMS R.W.: *Microlumbar discectomy. Surgical techniques.* Randolp. M.A. Codman and Shurtleff, 1977.

WILLIAMS R.W.: Microlumbar discectomy. *Spine*, 3, 175-182, 1978.

WILLIAMS R.W.: Microlumbar discectomy. A 12- year statistical review. *Spine*, **11**, 851-852, 1986.

WILSON D.H.: Microsurgical lumbar discectomy: preliminary report of 83 consecutive cases. *Neurosurg.*, **4**, 137, 1979.

WILSON D.H.: Microsurgical and standard removal of the protruded lumbar disc. *Neurosurg.*, **8**, 422, 1981.

YASARGIL M.G.: *Microsurgical operation of herniated lumbar disc. Advances in neurosurgery*, vol. 5, Springer - Verlag, Berlin - Heidelberg - New York, 1977.

ZEIGER H.E.: Microsurgical lumbar discectomy. *Alabama Med.*, **6**, 1983.